WE ARE ALL CANNIBALS

EUROPEAN PERSPECTIVES

For a complete list of books in the series, see pages 157–59.

Claude Lévi-Strauss

WITH A FOREWORD BY MAURICE OLENDER

TRANSLATED BY JANE MARIE TODD

WE ARE ALL CANNIBALS

And Other Essays

COLUMBIA UNIVERSITY PRESS ▲ NEW YORK

COLUMBIA UNIVERSITY PRESS

Publishers Since 1893

New York   Chichester, West Sussex

Copyright © 2013 Éditions du Seuil

Collection La Librairie du XXIme siècle, sous la direction de Maurice Olender

English translation © 2016 Columbia University Press

All rights reserved

This work received the French Voices Award for excellence in publication and translation. French Voices is a program created and funded by the French Embassy in the United States and FACE (French American Cultural Exchange).

Library of Congress Cataloging-in-Publication Data

Names: Lévi-Strauss, Claude, author. | Todd, Jane Marie, 1957– translator.
Title: We are all cannibals and other essays / Claude Lévi-Strauss ; with a foreword by Maurice Olender ; translated by Jane Marie Todd.
Other titles: Nous sommes tous des cannibales. English
Description: New York : Columbia University Press, 2016. | Series: European perspectives: a series in social thought and cultural criticism
Identifiers: LCCN 2015024328 | ISBN 9780231170680 (cloth) | ISBN 9780231541268 (e-book)
Subjects: LCSH: Structural anthropology.
Classification: LCC GN362 .L472513 2016 | DDC 301—dc23
LC record available at http://lccn.loc.gov/2015024328

Columbia University Press books are printed on permanent and durable acid-free paper.

This book is printed on paper with recycled content.

Printed in the United States of America

c 10 9 8 7 6 5 4 3 2

COVER DESIGN: CHANG JAE LEE

References to Internet Web sites (URLs) were accurate at the time of writing. Neither the author nor Columbia University Press is responsible for URLs that may have expired or changed since the manuscript was prepared.

CONTENTS

v

FOREWORD

Maurice Olender

Claude Lévi-Strauss composed the pages collected in this volume at the request of *La Repubblica*, a major Italian daily newspaper. The result: a set of sixteen original texts written in French between 1989 and 2000.

In each case Lévi-Strauss, taking a current event as his starting point, tackles some of the major debates of the time. Whether he is discussing the mad cow disease epidemic, different forms of cannibalism (alimentary or therapeutic), or racial prejudice linked to ritual practices such as female excision and male circumcision, the ethnologist helps us understand the social phenomena unfolding before our eyes. In doing so, he evokes Montaigne's writings, one of the founding monuments of Western modernity: "Everyone gives the title of barbarism to everything that is not in use in his own country" (1.31, Charles Cotton translation).

Lévi-Strauss points out that any practice, any belief or custom, "however bizarre, shocking, or even revolting it may appear," can be explained only within its own context. On the occasion of the four hundredth anniversary of Montaigne's death in 1992, the anthropologist revived a philosophical debate that is still current: "On the one hand, the philosophy of the Enlightenment subjects all historical societies to its criticism and cherishes the utopian dream of a rational society. On the other, relativism rejects any absolute criterion by which a culture could allow itself to judge different cultures. Since Montaigne, and following his example, we have never stopped looking for a way out of that contradiction."

Like all Claude Lévi-Strauss's writings, this volume, whose title is taken from one of its chapters, emphasizes the inextricable link between "mythic thought and scientific thought" but without reducing one to the other. He recalls that between so-called complex societies and those wrongly designated "primitive or archaic," there is not the great distance long imagined to exist. That observation arises from a mode of proceeding—in other words, from a method—that also aspires to be an intelligible approach to the everyday: "The faraway illuminates the near, but the near can also illuminate the faraway."

That sort of observation, that practice of the gaze in which the near and the faraway illuminate each other, was already in place in 1952, in "Santa Claus Burned as a Heretic," originally written for *Les Temps modernes* and reprinted as part 1 of this volume. In this article about a recent ritual that had emerged in the West, Lévi-Strauss writes: "It is not every day that the ethnologist finds the occasion to observe in his own society the sudden growth of a rite and even of a cult." He is cautious, however, immediately adding that it is both easier and more difficult to understand our own societies: "Easier, because the continuity of experience is maintained in all its moments and in each of its nuances; more difficult as well, because it is on such occasions, only too rare, that one realizes the extreme complexity of even the most tenuous social transformations."

In these newspaper columns, which bear the stamp of the last years of the twentieth century, we again find the lucidity and tonic pessimism of the great anthropologist. Translated into some thirty languages, his work now marks the beginning of our twenty-first century.

WE ARE ALL CANNIBALS

PART I

SANTA CLAUS BURNED AS A HERETIC

1952

In France, the Christmas holidays of 1951 were marked by a controversy that seems to have deeply affected the press and the general public, and which introduced a rare sour note into the usually joyous atmosphere of that time of year. For several months the church authorities, speaking through certain prelates, had been expressing their disapproval of the growing importance that families and merchants were granting to the figure of Santa Claus. They denounced a worrisome "paganization" of the Feast of the Nativity, which turned thoughts away from the properly Christian meaning of the celebration, in favor of a myth without religious value. These attacks increased as Christmas approached. More discreetly no doubt, but just as firmly, the Protestant churches joined their voices to that of the Catholic Church. Letters from readers and articles in newspapers, from various perspectives but generally hostile to the church's position, have already attested to the interest sparked by that affair. It reached a climax on December 24 at an event that the correspondent for *France-Soir* reported in the following words:

In front of the children of the church's boys and girls clubs
Santa Claus was burned on the square
outside the cathedral of Dijon
Dijon, December 24 (dispatch *France-Soir*)

Santa Claus was hanged yesterday afternoon from the gates of the cathedral of Dijon and publicly burned on the parvis. That spectacular execution unfolded in the presence of hundreds of children from the church's boys and girls clubs. The decision was made with the agreement of the clergy, who condemned Santa Claus as a usurper and a heretic. He was accused of paganizing the Christmas holiday and of installing himself like a cuckoo in another bird's nest, taking up more and more space. He is reproached especially for having introduced himself into all the public schools, from which the nativity scene is scrupulously banned.

Sunday at three o'clock P.M., the unfortunate white-bearded fellow, like many innocents, paid for a sin for which those who will applaud his execution are guilty. The fire set his beard ablaze, and he vanished in the smoke.

A press release was issued after the execution. Here is the gist:

Representing all Christian homes in the parish who wish to fight lies, two hundred and fifty children who had gathered in front of the main door of the cathedral of Dijon burned Santa Claus.

This was not entertainment but a symbolic gesture. Santa Claus was sacrificed as a burnt offering. If the truth be known, lies cannot awaken religious feelings in the child and are by no means a method of education. Let others say and write what they like; let them see Father Christmas as a counterweight to Father Flog.[1]

As for those of us who are Christians, the Christmas holiday must remain the anniversary of the birth of the Savior.

The execution of Santa Claus on the square outside the cathedral was judged in many different ways by the general population and elicited sharp comments even from Catholics.

Furthermore, that inopportune event may well have consequences unforeseen by its organizers.

The affair has divided the city into two camps.

Dijon is awaiting the resurrection of Santa Claus, murdered yesterday on the cathedral parvis. At six o'clock tonight, he will rise from the dead at city hall. An official press release announced that, like every other year, Santa Claus was asking the children of Dijon to come to Place de la Libération, and that he would speak to them from the rooftop of city hall, where he will make his way under the spotlights.

The canon Kir, deputy and mayor of Dijon, is said to have refrained from choosing sides in this delicate affair.

The same day, Santa Claus's fate was at the top of the news: not a single newspaper failed to comment on the incident, some—such as *France-Soir,* the largest-circulation newspaper in France—even went so far as to devote their editorial to it. In general, the attitude of the Dijon clergy met with disapproval; so much so, it seems, that the religious authorities judged it wise to beat a retreat or, at the very least, to observe a discreet silence. It is said, however, that our state ministers are divided on the question. The tone of most of the articles is one of tactful sentimentality: it is so nice to believe in Santa Claus, it doesn't do anyone any harm, children derive great satisfaction from it and store up delightful memories for their adult years, and so on. But the articles are evading the question rather than responding to it: the issue is not to explain why children are fond of Santa Claus but rather why adults were impelled to invent him. In any event, these reactions are so generally shared that there can be no doubt that public opinion and the church are at odds on this point. Despite the inconsequentiality of the incident, that discord is important because a gradual reconciliation has been occurring in France since the end of the Occupation, between the public, unbelievers for the most part, and religion. The accession to government councils by a political party as religiously oriented as the Mouvement Républicain Populaire is clearly evidence of that. The traditional anticlerical wing has seized the unhoped-for opportunity offered them: it is that group, in Dijon and elsewhere, that suddenly made itself the protector of our threatened Santa Claus. What a paradox: Santa Claus as symbol of irreligion! In this instance, it is as if the church were adopting a critical attitude, eagerly pursuing frankness and truth, even as the rationalists have become the guardians of superstition. That apparent reversal of roles is sufficient to suggest that this innocent affair conceals more profound realities. We have before us a symptomatic manifestation of a very rapid evolution in mores and beliefs, in France in the first place, but no doubt elsewhere as well. It is not every day that the ethnologist finds the occasion to observe in his own society the sudden growth of a rite and even of a cult; to seek its causes and to study its impact on the other forms of religious life; and finally, to try to understand to what general transformations, mental and social, these visible manifestations are linked. The church, with its wealth of traditional experience in these matters, was not wrong about these manifestations, at least insofar as it attributed a significant value to them.

*

* *

For about the last three years, ever since economic activity has returned almost to normal, the celebration of Christmas in France has taken on a magnitude unknown before the war. It is certain that this development, both in its material importance and in the forms it takes, is a direct result of the influence and prestige of the United States of America. Large fir trees, illuminated at night, have been put up at intersections and on the main avenues; fancy Christmas wrapping paper has gone on sale, as have greeting cards with pictures on them, accompanied by the practice of displaying them on the recipient's mantel during the crucial week; the Salvation Army hangs its kettles on squares and in the streets, soliciting contributions; and in department stores, individuals dressed up as Santa Claus listen to children's pleas. All these practices, which even a few years ago appeared puerile and odd to French people visiting the United States—some of the most obvious signs of the fundamental incompatibility between our two mentalities—have taken root and become acclimatized in

France with an ease and ubiquity that are a lesson for the historian of civilization to ponder.

In that realm and in others, we are witnessing an instance of diffusion on a vast scale, not very different no doubt from those archaic phenomena we were accustomed to study, based on the remote examples of the fire piston or the outrigger canoe. But it is both easier and more difficult to think rationally about events that unfold before our eyes and for which our own society is the theater. Easier, because the continuity of experience is maintained with all its moments and each of its nuances; more difficult as well, because it is on such occasions, only too rare, that one realizes the extreme complexity of even the most tenuous social transformations; and because the apparent reasons we attribute to events in which we are actors are very different from the real causes that assign us a role in them.

It would be too simple, then, to explain the development of the Christmas celebration in France solely in terms of the influence of the United States. Borrowings exist, but the reasons for their existence are only very incompletely contained within them. Let me give a quick list of the obvious ones: there are now more Americans living in France, and they celebrate Christmas in their accustomed manner; films, digests, and American novels, and also some reports in the major newspapers have made American customs better known here, and they enjoy the prestige attached to the military and economic might of the United States; it is also not impossible that the Marshall Plan directly or indirectly favored the import of a few commodities associated with Christmas rituals. But all these factors are inadequate to explain the phenomenon. Customs imported from the United States are taking root even among strata of the population that are unaware of where these customs originated; and the working classes, for whom the Communist influence would seem to discredit anything bearing the label "Made in USA," are adopting them as readily as the others. In addition to diffusion alone, therefore, we must mention the important process that Alfred Kroeber—the first to identify it—called "stimulus diffusion." In such cases, the imported practice is not assimilated but rather plays the role of a catalyst; that is, by its mere presence, it gives rise to an analogous practice that was already present in its potential state in the secondary environment. Let me illustrate this point with an example directly touching on the subject at hand. The paper manufacturer who goes to the United States at the invitation of his American colleagues or on a business trip observes that special paper is produced there for Christmas wrappings. He borrows the idea: that is a diffusion phenomenon. The Parisian housewife goes to her neighborhood stationer's to buy the paper she needs to wrap her presents and, in the display window, sees paper that is prettier and better made than that with which she had formerly made do. She doesn't know a thing about the American custom, but that paper satisfies an aesthetic requirement and expresses an emotional inclination that was already present but had previously had no means of expression. In purchasing the paper, she (unlike the manufacturer) is not borrowing a foreign custom directly, but that custom, once acknowledged, leads her to adopt an identical one.

Furthermore, it must not be forgotten that even before the war, the celebration of Christmas was becoming more elaborate in France and throughout Europe. That development was linked in the first place to a gradual improvement in the standard of living, but it also had less obvious causes. Christmas in the form we know it is essentially a modern celebration, despite its many seemingly archaic characteristics. The use of mistletoe is not, at least not immediately, a druid survival, since it appears to have come back into fashion during the Middle Ages. Christmas trees are not mentioned anywhere prior to their appearance in certain seventeenth-century German texts. They reached England in the eighteenth century, France only in the nineteenth. In his dictionary, Émile Littré does not seem to have been well acquainted with them, or rather, they take a form there rather different from the one familiar to us. In the entry "Noël," he defines *sapin de Noël* as referring "in some countries to a fir or holly branch decorated in various ways, especially with candy and toys to give to children, who look forward to it with excitement." The diversity of names given to the personage whose role is to distribute the toys—"Father Christmas," "Saint Nicholas," "Santa Claus"—also shows that he is the product of a phenomenon of convergence and not an ancient prototype preserved everywhere.

But modern developments invent nothing: they simply recompose from bits and pieces an old celebration whose importance is never completely forgotten. For Littré, the Christmas tree is an almost exotic institution; but significantly, Chéruel notes in his *Dictionnaire historique des institutions, moeurs et coutumes de la France* (*Historical Dictionary of Institutions, Mores, and Customs of France*)—a reworking, as the author himself admits, of Sainte-Palaye's dictionary of national antiquities (1697–1781)—"Christmas . . . was for several centuries, and *until recently* [my emphasis], an occasion for family festivities." A description follows of Christmas festivities in the thirteenth century, which appear to have been in every way equal to our own. We are thus in the presence of a ritual whose importance has fluctuated a great deal over history, with peaks and valleys. The American form is only the most modern of these incarnations.

Incidentally, these brief comments suffice to show how wary we must be, in dealing with problems of this kind, about giving overly simplistic explanations by automatically appealing to "vestiges" and "survivals." If there had never been a cult of trees in prehistoric times, one that has continued in various folk customs, modern Europe would undoubtedly not have "invented" the Christmas tree. And, as I demonstrated above, it is actually a recent invention. Yet that invention did not arise out of nowhere. Other medieval customs are perfectly well attested: the Yule log (which in Paris became a cake, the *bûche de Noël*) made of a trunk big enough to burn all night long; Christmas candles, large enough to achieve the same result; and the decoration of buildings with verdant branches of ivy, holly, and fir (dating back to the Roman Saturnalia, to which I shall return). Finally, and completely unrelated to Christmas, the romances of the knights of the Round Table speak of a supernatural tree completely covered in lights. In that context, the Christmas tree appears to be a syncretic solution—that is, one that concentrates in a single object requirements previously fulfilled piecemeal: magic tree, fire, long-lasting light, evergreens. By contrast, Santa Claus in his present form is a modern creation; even more recent is the belief that he lives at the North Pole, which is to say, in Greenland, and travels in a sled hitched to a team of reindeer. (Greenland being a Danish possession, that belief has obliged Denmark to maintain a special post office to reply to letters from children all over the world.) It is said that this aspect of the legend developed for the most part during World War II, when U.S. troops were stationed in Iceland and Greenland. And yet the reindeer are not there by chance: English documents dating to the Renaissance mention reindeer trophies paraded about during Christmas dances, prior to any belief in Santa Claus and a fortiori to the formation of his legend.

Very old elements are thus shuffled and reshuffled, new ones introduced; original forms are discovered for perpetuating, transforming, or reviving ancient practices. There is nothing specifically new about what could be called, no pun intended, the rebirth of Christmas. Why, then, does it stir such emotions, and why does some of the animosity focus on the figure of Santa Claus?

*
* *

Santa Claus is dressed in scarlet; he is a king. His white beard, his furs and boots, and the sled on which he travels evoke winter. He is called "Father Christmas" and is an old man: he therefore incarnates the authority of the elders in its benevolent form. All that is fairly clear, but where should he be placed within religious typology? He is not a mythical being, since there is no myth that accounts for his origin and functions; and he is not a legendary figure, because no quasi-historical narrative is attached to him. In fact, that supernatural and immutable being, eternally fixed in form and defined by a single function and a periodic return, belongs rather to the family of deities. He is worshiped by children at certain times of the year, through letters and supplications; he rewards those who are nice and withholds from those who are naughty. He is the god of an age cohort in our society (an age cohort, in fact, that can be adequately defined by the belief in Santa Claus), and the only difference between Santa Claus and a genuine god is that adults do not believe in him, though they encourage their children to believe and sustain that belief by means of a large number of deceptions.

Thus Santa Claus is in the first place the expression of the differential status between small children on the one hand, adolescents and adults on the other. In that respect, he is linked to a vast set of beliefs and practices that ethnologists have studied in most societies, namely, rites of passage and initiation. There are few human groups in which, in one form or another, children (and sometimes also women) are not excluded from the society of men by virtue of their ignorance of certain mysteries or their belief—carefully nurtured—in a few illusions that the adults reserve the right to unveil at the opportune moment, thus sanctioning the aggregation of the younger generation to their own. Sometimes these rites bear an astonishing resemblance to those we are examining at the moment. How can we not be struck, for example, by the similarity between Santa Claus and the kachinas of Native Americans in the southwestern United States? These costumed and masked figures incarnate gods and ancestors; they return periodically to visit the village, to dance and to punish or reward the children, since arrangements are made to ensure that the children will not recognize their parents or loved ones in their traditional disguises. Santa Claus certainly belongs to the same family, though secondary players are now relegated to the background: the bogeyman, Father Flog, and so on. It is extremely significant that the same child-rearing principles that currently proscribe calling on these punitive "kachinas" have led to the glorification of the benevolent figure of Santa Claus. That is, Santa Claus has not been included in the same condemnation, as the development of positive and rationalist thought might have led us to expect. In that regard, there has been no rationalization of child-rearing methods, since Santa Claus is no more "rational" than Father Flog (the church is right on that point). Rather, we are witnessing a displacement of the myth, and that is what needs to be explained.

It is quite certain that rites and myths of initiation have a practical function in human societies: they help elders keep youngsters well-behaved and obedient. Throughout the year, we invoke Santa Claus to remind children that his generosity will be meted out on the basis of how good they are. And the periodic nature of the distribution of gifts serves the purpose of keeping children's demands in check, reducing to a brief period the time when they actually have the *right* to demand gifts. But that simple statement is sufficient to shatter the traditional parameters of the utilitarian explanation. For how is it that children have rights and that these rights are imposed so imperiously on adults that they are obliged to elaborate a costly and complicated mythology and ritual in order to contain them? Right away we see that the belief in Santa Claus is not only a *hoax* playfully inflicted on children by adults; to a very great extent, it is the result of a very expensive *transaction* between the two generations. The ritual as a whole is like the green plants—fir, holly, ivy, mistletoe—with which we decorate our homes. Although they are now a gratuitous luxury, they were once, in a few regions at least, the object of an *exchange* between two classes of the population. In England on Christmas Eve, even into the late eighteenth century, women went "a-gooding," that is, they begged from house to house and provided donors with small green branches in return. We find children in a similar bargaining position, and it is useful to note here that children sometimes disguised themselves as women to beg from Saint Nicholas. Women and children both are uninitiated.

Yet there is a very important aspect of the initiation rituals to which adequate attention has not always been paid, one that sheds even more light on their nature than the utilitarian considerations mentioned previously. Take the example of the kachina ritual of the Pueblo Indians. Are children kept in ignorance of the human identity of the individuals who incarnate the kachinas so that the youngsters will fear and respect them and will therefore behave? Yes, no doubt, but that is only a secondary function of the ritual. As it happens, there is another explanation, which the original myth perfectly illuminates. That myth explains that kachinas are the souls of the first indigenous children, who drowned tragically in a river during the ancestral migrations. Kachinas are thus both proof of death and evidence of life after death. But there is more: when the ancestors of the present-day Indians had finally settled in their village, the myth says, the kachinas came every year to pay them a visit and, when they left, they took the children with them. The indigenous people, in despair about losing their progeny, obtained a pledge from the kachinas that they would remain in the next world in exchange for the promise that the villagers would represent them every year with masks and dances. If children are excluded from the mystery of the kachinas, therefore, it is not in the first place so that they will be intimidated. I would rather say it is for the opposite reason: it is because the children *are* kachinas. They are kept at a remove from the hoax because they represent the reality in relation to which the hoax constitutes a sort of compromise. Their place is elsewhere: not with the masks and the living but with the gods and the dead, with the gods, who *are* the dead. And the dead are children.

I believe this interpretation can be extended to all rites of initiation and even to all occasions when society divides itself into two groups. "Non-initiation" is not purely a state of privation defined by ignorance, illusion, or other negative elements. The relationship between initiates and the uninitiated has a positive content. It is a complementary relationship between two groups, one of which represents the dead and the other the living. In the course of the ritual itself, the roles are often reversed, several times in fact, since duality gives rise to a reciprocity of perspectives that—like the images in mirrors placed opposite each other—may repeat themselves ad infinitum. If the uninitiated are the dead, they are also super-initiates; and if, as often happens as well, it is the initiates who personify the ghosts of the dead to terrify the novices, it will be the novices who, in a later stage of the ritual, will be called upon to disperse them and prevent their return. Without pursuing any further these considerations, which would take us far from the matter at hand, I simply recall that, inasmuch as the rites and beliefs associated with Santa Claus belong to a sociology of initiation (and there is no doubt about that), they bring to light, behind the opposition between children and adults, a more profound opposition between the dead and the living.

*
* *

We have arrived at this conclusion by means of a purely synchronic analysis of the function of certain rituals and the content of the myths that serve as their foundation. But a diachronic analysis would have led to the same result. Generally speaking, historians of religion and folklorists acknowledge that the distant origins of Santa Claus are found in the Abbas Stultorum, the "Abbot of Unreason" or "Lord of Misrule." For a certain span of time, these figures were kings of Christmas; they are recognized as being the heirs of the king of the Saturnalia in the Roman period. Now Saturnalia was the feast of the *larvae,* that is, of those who had died violently or had been left unburied. And behind old man Saturn, devourer of children, can be glimpsed a series of symmetrical images: Father Christmas, benefactor of children; the Scandinavian Yule goat, a horned demon from the underworld who bears gifts for children; Saint Nicholas, who brings children back to life and showers them with presents; and finally, the kachinas, children who died prematurely, who renounce their role as child killers to become dispensers, by turns, of punishments and gifts. In addition, like the kachinas, the archaic prototype of Saturn is a god of germination. In fact, the modern figure of Santa Claus or Father Christmas appeared as a result of a syncretic fusion of several figures: the Abbot of Unreason; the child bishop chosen in the name of Saint Nicholas; and Saint Nicholas himself, since beliefs relating to stockings, shoes, and chimneys hark back to his feast. The Abbot of Unreason ruled on December 25; the Feast of Saint Nicholas took place on December 6; and the child bishops were chosen on the Feast of the Holy Innocents, that is, on December 28. Scandinavian Yule was celebrated in December as well. We are led directly back to the *libertas decembris* of which Horace speaks and which, already in the eighteenth century, du Tillot invoked to link Christmas to Saturnalia.

Explanations in terms of survivals are always incomplete since customs do not disappear or survive for no reason. When they live on, the cause is to be found less in the sluggishness of historical change than in the permanence of a function that an analysis of the present ought to reveal to us. I have given the Pueblo Indians a predominant place in my discussion precisely because the absence of any conceivable historical relationship between their institutions and our own (with the exception of certain late Spanish influences in the seventeenth century) demonstrates well that, with the rites of Christmas, we are in the presence not only of historical vestiges but of forms of thought and behaviors that belong to the most general conditions of life in society. Saturnalia and the medieval celebration of Christmas do not contain the ultimate explanation for a ritual that is otherwise inexplicable and meaningless; they provide comparative material useful for extracting the profound meaning of recurrent institutions.

It is not surprising that the non-Christian aspects of the Christmas holiday resemble Saturnalia. Indeed, there are good reasons to believe that the church set the date of the Nativity on December 25 (instead of in March or January) in order to substitute its commemoration for the pagan feasts that had originally occurred on December 17 but which, by the end of the Empire, had come to extend over seven days, that is, until the 24th. In fact, from antiquity to the Middle Ages, the "December holidays" always displayed the same characteristics: first, the decoration of buildings with green plants; then, gifts exchanged or given to children, followed by gaiety and feasting; and finally, fraternization between rich and poor, masters and servants.

When the facts are analyzed more closely, certain structural similarities, equally striking, come to light. Like the Roman Saturnalia, medieval Christmas displayed two syncretic and opposing traits. In the first place, it was a gathering together and a communion. The distinctions between classes and conditions were temporarily abolished: slaves or servants sat at the master's table, and the master became their domestic; the well-stocked tables were open to all; men and women swapped clothing. At the same time, however, the social group was split in two: young people formed into an autonomous body, elected a ruler, the Abbot of Youth, or, in Scotland, the Abbot of Unreason; and, as that title indicates, they engaged in unreasonable behavior, committed abuses against the rest of the population. We know that, until the Renaissance, these could take the most extreme forms: blasphemy, theft, rape, even murder. At Christmastime, as during Saturnalia, society's functioning followed a dual rhythm of *increased solidarity* and *exacerbated antagonism*, and these two characteristics were presented as a pair of correlative opposites. The figure of the Abbot of Unreason established a mediation of sorts between these two aspects. He was acknowledged and even enthroned by the regular authorities; his mission was to issue the order for the excesses even while containing them within certain limits. What relationship is there between that figure and his function and the figure and function of his distant descendant Santa Claus?

It is imperative to distinguish carefully between the historical perspective and the structural perspective. Historically, as I said, the Santa Claus of Western Europe and his predilection for chimneys and stockings are the result pure and simple of a recent displacement of the Feast of Saint Nicholas, which was assimilated to the Christmas celebration occurring three weeks later. That explains why the young abbot became an old man—but only in part, since the transformations are more systematic than the randomness of historical connections and proximity on the calendar would allow us to admit. A real figure became a mythical figure; a manifestation of youth symbolizing antagonism toward adults was transformed into a symbol of maturity expressing benevolent tendencies toward young people; the apostle of bad behavior is now in charge of sanctioning good conduct. Adolescents openly aggressive toward their parents are replaced by parents concealing themselves behind false beards to satisfy the children. The imaginary mediator replaces the real mediator, and, even as he changes in nature, his function is reversed.

Let us immediately dismiss one type of consideration that, though not essential to the debate, runs the risk of perpetuating confusion. "Youth" as an age cohort has largely disappeared from contemporary society (in the last few years, we have seen certain attempts to reconstitute it, but it is too early to tell what the result will be). A ritual that was formerly divided among three groups of protagonists—small children, young people, and adults—now involves only two, at least as far as Christmas is concerned: adults and children. The "unreason" of Christmas has therefore largely lost its foothold; it has been displaced and at the same time attenuated. Within the adult group, it survives only as Christmas Eve celebrations at nightclubs and New Year's Eve on Times Square. But let us rather examine the role of children.

In the Middle Ages, children did not wait patiently for their toys to come down the chimney. Rather, "mummers"—generally a gang of children wearing disguises and called for that reason *guisarts* in Old French—went from house to house, singing and expressing their best wishes, for which they would receive fruit and cake in return. Significantly, they evoked death to assert their claims. In eighteenth-century Scotland, they sang this verse:

> Rise up, good wife, and be no' swier [lazy]
> To deal your bread as long's you're here;
> The time will come when you'll be dead,
> And neither want nor meal nor bread.[2]

Even if we did not have that valuable indication—and the no less significant information about the disguises that turned the actors into spirits or ghosts—we would have others at our disposal, taken from a study of the begging practices of children. We know this activity is not limited to Christmas.[3] It occurs throughout the entire critical period of autumn, when night threatens day and the dead stalk the living. Christmas begging began several weeks (generally three) before the Feast of the Nativity, thus establishing the connection with the begging, also in costume, of the Feast of Saint Nicholas, named after the man who brought dead children back to life. The nature of this custom is even better marked by the first instance of begging during this season, on All Hallows' Eve, which by ecclesiastic decision came to fall on the night before All Saints' Day. Even today in English-speaking countries, children dressed up as ghosts and skeletons persecute adults, unless they purchase their peace and quiet with little treats. The advance of autumn, from its beginning until the winter solstice—which brings the relief of light and life—is thus accompanied at the ritual level by a dialectical procedure whose principal stages are: (1) the return of the dead; (2) threatening and persecutory conduct on their part; (3) the establishment of a modus vivendi with the living, which consists of an exchange of services and presents; and (4) the triumph of life on Christmas, when the dead, showered with gifts, leave the living in peace until the following autumn. It is revealing that until the last century, Latin and Catholic countries placed the emphasis on the Feast of Saint Nicholas, that is, on the most restrained form of the relationship, whereas the Anglo-Saxon countries tended to split it into two extreme and antithetical forms: Halloween, when children play the role of the dead to extort treats from the adults; and Christmas, when adults fulfill the wishes of children in order to glory in their vitality.

The apparently contradictory characteristics of Christmas rites are thereby resolved: for three months, the visitations of the dead among the living had become increasingly insistent and oppressive. On the day they took their leave, it was therefore permitted to celebrate them and provide them with one last opportunity to manifest themselves freely or, as English so felicitously puts it, "to raise hell." And who can personify the dead in a society of the living if not all those who in one way or another are incompletely integrated into the group; that is, who partake of *alterity*, the very mark of that supreme dualism between the dead and the living? It should therefore come as no surprise that strangers, slaves, and children become the principal beneficiaries of the holiday. In that respect, an inferior political or social condition and a lack of adult status serve as equivalent criteria. There is no end of evidence, in fact, especially for Scandinavia and the Slavic countries, that Christmas Eve dinner is by its very nature a meal offered to the dead: the guests play the role of the dead, children that of angels, and angels themselves that of the dead. It is therefore no surprise that Christmas and New Year's (its twin) are gift-giving holidays: the feast of the dead is essentially the feast of the Other, since the fact of being other is the first approximate image we are able to form of the dead.

We are now in a position to provide an answer to one of the questions raised at the beginning of this study. Why did the figure of Santa Claus develop, and why does the church regard that development with anxiety?

We have seen that Santa Claus is the heir, as well as the antithesis, of the Lord of Misrule or the Abbot of Unreason. That transformation is in the first place the sign of an improvement in our relations with death: we no longer judge it useful, in order to clear our accounts with death, to allow it periodically to subvert law and order. These relations are now dominated by a somewhat disdainful spirit of benevolence: we can be generous, take the initiative, since it is now simply a matter of offering death gifts and even toys—that is, symbols. But that attenuation in the relations between the dead and the living does not come at the expense of the personage who incarnates it: on the contrary, it seems he only becomes the stronger. The contradiction would be irresolvable were we not to concede that a different attitude toward death continues to make inroads among our contemporaries. It consists not of the traditional fear of spirits and ghosts perhaps but rather fear of everything that death represents in itself and also in life: depletion, scarcity, hardship. Let us venture to consider the tender care we take of Santa Claus, the precautions and sacrifices we agree to make to keep his prestige intact among children. Is it not because deep down we still harbor the desire to believe, however little, in a boundless generosity, a kindness without ulterior motives, a brief interval during which all fear, all envy, and all bitterness are suspended? No doubt we cannot fully share the illusion, but what justifies our efforts is that, fostered in others, it provides us with at least the opportunity to warm ourselves by the flame lit in those young souls. The belief we promote in our children, namely, that their toys come from a supernatural world, provides us with an alibi for the secret impulse that incites us to offer them to the supernatural world on the pretext of giving them to children. By that means, Christmas gifts remain a true sacrifice to the delight of being alive, which consists in the first place of not dying.

Salomon Reinach once wrote, with a great deal of insight, that the major difference between ancient and modern religions is that "pagans prayed to the dead, whereas Christians pray for the dead."[4] It is undoubtedly a long way from prayers to the dead and the prayer, entangled with apotropaism, that every year and increasingly we address to little children—traditional incarnations of the dead—so that by believing in Santa Claus they will consent to help us believe in life. We have, however, disentangled the threads that attest to the continuity between these two expressions of a single reality. But the church is certainly not wrong when it denounces the belief in Santa Claus as the most solid bastion and one of the most active sites of paganism in modern humankind. It remains to be seen whether moderns as well can defend their right to be pagan.

In conclusion, one final remark: it is a long journey from the king of Saturnalia to Santa Claus. Along the way, an essential trait—the most archaic perhaps—of the former seems to have been permanently lost. Frazer showed long ago that the king of Saturnalia is himself the heir of an ancient prototype. This individual, having personified King Saturn and been allowed every excess for a month's time, was solemnly sacrificed on the altar of the god. Thanks to the auto-da-fé of Dijon, therefore, that hero is reconstituted with all his characteristics, and it is not the least of the paradoxes in this odd affair that, in wanting to put an end to Santa Claus, the Dijon ecclesiastics merely restored in his plenitude, after an eclipse of several millennia, a ritual figure whose enduring nature they themselves ended up demonstrating on the pretext of destroying it.

PART 2

WE ARE ALL CANNIBALS

1989-2002

1

"TOPSY-TURVYDOM"

Nearly twenty-five hundred years ago, Herodotus, on visiting Egypt, was astonished by practices that were at odds with those he had been able to observe elsewhere. The Egyptians, he wrote, behave in all things contrary to other peoples. Not only do the women engage in trade while the men remain at home and weave, but the men begin the weft at the bottom of the loom, not at the top as in other countries. The women urinate standing up, the men squat. I shall not go on with the list.

Closer to our own time, in the late nineteenth century the English-man Basil Hall Chamberlain, a longtime professor at the University of Tokyo, gave the title "Topsy-Turvydom" to an entry in his book *Things Japanese*, which takes the form of a dictionary. As he explained, "the Japanese do many things in a way that runs directly counter to Euro-pean ideas of what is natural and proper. To the Japanese themselves our ways appear equally unaccountable." A series of examples fol-lows, echoing those cited by Herodotus twenty-four centuries earlier in reference to a different country, similarly exotic in the eyes of his fellow citizens.

No doubt the examples Chamberlain provided are not all equally convincing. Japanese writing is not the only one in the world that is read from right to left. It is not only in Japan that the address on a letter gives the name of the city first, then the street and house number, and finally, the name of the addressee. The difficulties that dressmakers during the Meiji period had when trimming European-style dresses do not necessarily reveal a trait of the national character. By contrast, it is striking that these same dressmakers threaded their needles by pushing the eye over the thread, which was held still, instead of pushing the thread into the eye; and that, while sewing, they pushed the fabric onto the needle instead of sticking the needle into the fabric, as we do. The ancient Japanese mounted their horses from the right and backed their animals into the barn.

Foreign visitors are astonished that Japanese carpenters saw by pulling the tool toward them and not by pushing it away as we do, and that they similarly manipulate their "drawknife," a two-handled knife used for planing and thinning out wood. In Japan, the potter sets the wheel in motion with his left foot, clockwise, unlike the European or Chinese potter, who sets it in motion with his right foot, counterclockwise.

Indeed, these practices do not simply differentiate Japan from Europe: the line of demarcation runs between insular Japan and continental Asia. In addition to many other elements, Japan borrowed from Chinese culture the crosscut saw, which cuts by pushing; but from the fourteenth century on, saws that cut by pulling, invented in Japan itself, supplanted the Chinese model. And the drawknife that is pushed, which came from China in the sixteenth century, gave way a hundred years later to models that the user pulls toward himself. How are we to explain the characteristic that all these innovations have in common?

We might attempt to solve the problem case by case. Japan has little iron ore, and a saw that is pulled requires a thinner piece of metal than the other kind: reasons of economy, therefore. But would the same argument be valid for the drawknife? And how could it be applied to the different ways of threading a needle and of sewing, which, however, proceed on the same principle? To find a specific explanation in each instance, we would have to engage in extravagant flights of the imagination, and we would never be done with it.

A general explanation comes to mind. If, in the work they perform, Japanese men and women move toward the self, inward and not outward, is it not because of their predilection for squatting, which allows them to reduce their furniture to the bare minimum? In the absence of workshop furniture, the artisan must support himself. The explanation appears so simple that it has been invoked not only for Japan but also for other regions of the world where similar observations have been made.

In the mid-nineteenth century, J. G. Swan, a prosperous Boston merchant who decided one day to abandon his family and (as Gauguin would later do) seek primitive simplicity far from home, noted that the Native Americans of the Pacific Northwest in the United States, already very acculturated in their use of knives, always cut toward themselves, as we do to cut a quill pen, he said, and did their work squatting on the ground whenever they had the opportunity. There is no question that there is a connection between one's working posture and the way of handling a tool. It remains to be seen, however, if one explains the other—and if so, which one?—or if these two aspects of a single phenomenon have a common origin we might discover.

A Japanese friend and seasoned traveler told me one day that, in every city she visited, she could assess the ambient pollution by inspecting her husband's shirt collars. No Western woman, it seems to me, would follow that line of reasoning. Instead, she would think that her husband's neck was unclean. She would attribute an external effect to an internal cause: her reasoning would move from the inside outward. My Japanese friend reasoned from the outside inward, performing in her mind the same movement as, in Japanese practice, the dressmaker threading a needle, the carpenter sawing or planing wood.

Nothing sheds more light on the common reasons behind the little facts to which I have drawn attention than this example. Western thought is centrifugal; Japanese, centripetal. That is already clear in the language used by a cook. Unlike us, she does not "plunge" something into the frying oil but rather "lifts," "draws out," or "withdraws" (*ageru*) it from the oil. It is clear, more generally, in the syntax of the Japanese language, which constructs sentences by means of successive determiners, moving from the general to the specific, and places the subject at the end. The Japanese, when they leave home, will often say something like *itte mairimasu*, "going away I come back," a locution in which *itte*, the gerund of the verb *ikimasu*, reduces the act of going out to a circumstance in which the primary intention is to return. And it is true that, in ancient Japanese literature, journeys appear to be painful experiences that wrest one away from that "interior," *uchi*, to which one always yearns to return.

Western philosophers contrast Far Eastern thought to their own by noting two different attitudes toward the notion of the subject. In various ways, Hinduism, Taoism, and Buddhism all deny what for the West constitutes a fundamental and obvious fact: that of the self, whose illusory character these Eastern doctrines set out to demonstrate. For them, every being is only a precarious arrangement of biological and psychic phenomena, with no durable element such as a "self," merely an appearance destined to dissolve.

But Japanese thought is always original, and it distinguishes itself as much from the other Far Eastern philosophies as from our own. Unlike those philosophies, it does not annihilate the subject. Unlike Western philosophies, it refuses to make the self the obligatory starting point for any philosophical reflection, any project to reconstruct the world by means of thought. It has even been said that in a language such as Japanese, where the personal pronoun is used reluctantly, Descartes's maxim "I think, therefore I am" is rigorously untranslatable.

Instead of making the subject a cause, as we do, Japanese thought sees it rather as a result. The Western philosophy of the subject is centrifugal; that of Japan is centripetal, placing the subject at the end. That difference in mental attitudes is the same as what we saw lying just beneath the surface in the opposing ways of using tools: like the gestures the artisan performs toward himself, Japanese society makes self-consciousness an endpoint. It results from the manner in which increasingly small social and professional groups fit one into another. The counterpart to the Westerner's prejudice about autonomy is the constant need by the Japanese individual to define himself as a function of the group(s) to which he belongs, which he designates by the word *uchi.* That term means not only "house" but, within the house, the back room, in contrast to those leading to it or surrounding it.

The secondary and derivative reality that Japanese thought concedes to the self cannot provide the center toward which one tends and for which one yearns. Within a social and moral system thus conceived, there is no absolute order, such as the one China was able to ensure by means of an organized cult of ancestors and the exercise of filial piety. In Japan the elderly lose all authority and no longer count once they cease to be heads of families. In that area as well, the relative prevails over the absolute: family and society are perpetually shifting their focus. The distrust of theory (*tatemae*) and the primacy given to practice (*honne*) can be attributed to that deep-seated tendency.

But if Japanese life is dominated by a sense of relativity and impermanence, does that not imply that a certain sense of the absolute must find a place on the periphery of individual consciousness, to give consciousness a framework it does not have within itself? That may explain the role played in the modern history of Japan by the dogma of the divine origin of imperial power, the belief in racial purity, and the affirmation of a specificity of Japanese culture vis-à-vis other nations. To be viable, every system needs a certain rigidity, which may be internal or external to the elements composing it. Is it not partly because of that external rigidity, so disconcerting to Westerners because it reverses their way of conceiving the relation between the individual and his surroundings, that Japan was able to overcome the ordeals suffered during the nineteenth and twentieth centuries and to find, in the flexibility preserved within individual consciousnesses, a means for the successes it now enjoys?

2

IS THERE ONLY ONE TYPE

OF DEVELOPMENT?

Researchers have long wondered how a small, dispersed system of family agriculture like that practiced by present-day Maya farmers could have fed the hundreds or thousands of workers that had to be assembled onsite in pre-Columbian times to build the giant monuments of Mexico and Central America. The problem has become even more acute since the advent of archaeological excavations. They have taught us that Maya settlements were not simply royal residences or religious centers but true cities extending over several square kilometers and numbering tens of thousands of residents: lords, aristocrats, functionaries, servants, artisans. Where did their means of support come from?

In the last twenty years, aerial photography has begun to provide some answers. In Maya country and in some regions of South America that were formerly believed to have been occupied by very rustic societies, pictures taken from the air reveal the vestiges of astonishingly complex agricultural systems. One of them, in Colombia, covered over two hundred thousand hectares of floodplains. Between the beginning of the Christian era and the seventh century, thousands of drainage canals were dug; in between them, lands were cultivated on man-made embankments several hundred meters long, permanently irrigated and safeguarded from flooding. That intensive tuber-based agriculture, combined with fishing in the canals, could feed more than a thousand inhabitants per square kilometer.

On the banks of Lake Titicaca on the border between Peru and Bolivia, similar systems were recently discovered over an area of more than eighty thousand hectares. They had been in use between the first millennium BCE and the fifth century CE. Because of the arid climate and the long periods of frost due to altitude—the site is nearly four thousand meters above sea level—these zones are now only poor-quality grazing lands. The irrigation canals partly mitigated these climatic disadvantages. Their water kept things moist; in addition, it stored up heat during the day and released it slowly throughout the night, raising the ambient temperature by about two degrees. The tests done proved that these agricultural techniques would still be effective, and several Andean communities were persuaded to put them back into practice after centuries of disuse. The standard of living there improved considerably. Similar forms of intensive agriculture on a more modest scale existed and still exist in Melanesia and Polynesia.

Such observations oblige us to call into question the clear-cut distinction we are accustomed to make between so-called archaic societies and the rest. No doubt that first class of societies is not really "primitive": all societies have an equally long history behind them. But we believe ourselves justified in calling by that term those societies that survived until recent times whose declared ideal was to remain in the state in which the gods or ancestors had created them. They took measures to limit and regulate the size of their population and maintained an unchanging standard of living, which their social rules and metaphysical beliefs contributed toward protecting. Granted, these societies were not immune to change, but, to us at least, it seems that they differed from our own, which tolerate a perpetual disequilibrium. The idea prevails in our societies that one must struggle simply to survive, that one must gain new advantages every day so as not to lose those already acquired; and that time is a rare commodity of which there is never enough. Are we to conclude from this that the two types of society are incommensurable? In addition to the fact that farmers and artisans in so-called developed countries had until recently a vision of the world and of themselves not very different from that attributed to exotic peoples, the relationship between the two types of societies is actually more complex. We do not know a great deal about the long period—some two or three thousand years—at the beginning of which hominids made their appearance, but we are better informed about the last hundred thousand to two hundred thousand years. And everything shows that during that period technology did not evolve at a steady rate. The evolution was discontinuous; leaps forward and long periods of stagnation alternated with each other. Technological revolutions were localized in space and time. For hundreds of millennia humankind's ancestors confined themselves to selecting pebbles and making them sharp and easy to handle by chipping off flakes. With the "Levallois revolution" some two hundred thousand years ago, the technology became more complicated. Some fifteen distinct operations became necessary to process the block of flint in such a way that the flakes, used to manufacture tools of a determinate type, could be broken off with a stone hammer; then to refine these flakes with a hammer or bone needle. The flint pebble thus went from being a tool to being a raw material for making tools. "Blade" industries, which were even more economical in the use of material, coexisted with or replaced "flake-based" industries. Finally, the blades themselves became raw materials, broken into little pieces and fitted out with wooden or bone frames to make awls, arrowheads, saws, or sickles. These processes are called microlith industries.

There are sites in the Near East that are known to have been occupied continuously for tens of millennia, during which stone technologies and the form of tools did not change. By contrast, there were veritable technological explosions in prehistoric times, by both qualitative and quantitative measures.

In terms of quality, the most ancient jewelry known, dating to about the thirty-fifth millennium, came primarily from southwestern France but was made out of exotic materials imported from regions sometimes several hundred kilometers away. As for quantity, industrial ventures in the most modern sense of the term—though they date back to prehistoric times—are known to have existed in various parts of the world. They mass-produced certain types of objects or implements for the needs of the market. Intertribal fairs were held at the foot of the Pyrenees in southwestern France during the Magdalenian period, about fifteen thousand years ago. For sale there were seashells that had been imported from the Atlantic Ocean and the Mediterranean, tools carved in a flint of nonlocal provenance, and spear throwers mass-produced by the hundreds, in all likelihood. Examples of these launchers, all the same model, were discovered at sites more than 150 kilometers apart.

In Spiennes, Belgium, an underground flint operation riddled with mine shafts and galleries more than fifteen meters deep extended over about fifty hectares. It included specialized workshops, some to rough out the miners' picks and axes, others to give these implements their final form. In Grimes Cave in England, shafts by the hundreds allowed for the mining of thousands of cubic meters of chalk, from which flint nodules were extracted. In the protohistoric period, the mining and industrial center of Le Grand-Pressigny in the southern Loire Valley of France covered more than ten kilometers. It exported tools and weapons to as far away as Switzerland and Belgium; they were particularly valued because the color of the local flint resembled bronze. Stone imitations of metal weapons were thus being produced at a time when bronze was a costly material reserved for a minority.

Writing appeared in southern Mesopotamia in about 3400 BCE; for a millennium, it was used only to record merchandise inventories, tax revenues, land leases, and lists of offerings. It was not until about 2500 BCE that Mesopotamians began to transcribe myths, historical events, or texts we would call literary. All these examples show that a productivist mentality existed during various prehistoric and protohistoric eras and that it is not exclusive to the contemporary world.

Even peoples we consider archaic or backward were thus capable of mass-producing items as varied as stone tools, ceramic, and farm products, obtaining results that sometimes surpass our own. But that was not a gradual evolution always oriented in the same direction. Over the course of time, phases of rapid innovation were followed by periods of stagnation. Sometimes the two aspects even coexisted. There is not one type of evolution but a variety.

To understand that bewildering phenomenon, we may find inspiration in the thinking of certain biologists who challenge the hypothesis that the evolution of species comes about slowly and gradually, and that it retains from a multitude of small variations only those that offer a selective advantage, eliminating all the others. Plant or animal species can remain unchanged for hundreds of thousands, even millions of years. Individual variations within a population do not influence that stability: they offset one another and ultimately cancel one another out. By contrast, when changes affecting species do occur, they are very rapid (in geological time, that is); they probably come about when a few individuals find themselves isolated from the rest of their species, in a new environment to which they must adapt. Biological evolution, like technological evolution, occurs in fits and starts. Long periods of stasis are punctuated by short intervals during which massive changes occur (hence the name "punctualism" given to that theory). And that is not all: evolution, far from being homogeneous, assumes very different aspects depending on one's perspective: within a population, it manifests itself in slow and gradual variations; within the species, in transformations whose adaptive value is unclear; and within groups of species, in the form of a macroevolution, even though each species taken separately may not be subject to change for prolonged periods of time.

It is now acknowledged that modern man—*Homo sapiens sapiens*—appeared in the Near East, probably coming from Africa, about a hundred thousand years ago. But, based on the current state of our knowledge, we believe that his first aesthetic expressions (jewelry, sculpture, and engraved stones and bones) may not have appeared until sixty or seventy thousand years later—and they all appeared at once. Perhaps we ought to see this as an example of the "punctual" evolution known to biologists. So too the appearance in southwestern Europe fifteen to twenty thousand years ago of cave paintings of a dazzling perfection in, among other places, Altamira and Lascaux.

If the transposition of the punctualist hypothesis to human societies is legitimate, we would have to admit that the relationship between these societies and the environment, as reflected in their productive capacities and aesthetic expressions, has not always remained the same. We would have to give up the practice of placing human societies along a single continuum, classifying them as more or less developed. Rather, they would be seen to stem from heterogeneous models. And that is truly where the debates under way on the origin of agriculture lead.

*
* *

It was long believed that, apart from the industrial revolution that began in the nineteenth century, the production of consumable goods never increased so rapidly and so massively as it did with the invention of agriculture. Thanks to farming, it was thought, human groups were able to become sedentary and to assure themselves a regular supply of food by storing grain. The population increased; societies, now in possession of surpluses, had the luxury of supporting individuals or classes—leaders, nobles, priests, artisans—who did not participate in food production but performed specialized functions. Within the space of four or five millennia, the momentum provided and maintained by agriculture would have led human beings from a precarious way of life constantly threatened by famine to a stable existence, first in village communities, then in city-states, and finally in empires.

Such were until recently the prevailing views. But now that simple and grandiose reconstruction of human history is under attack. Detailed investigations of peoples without agriculture have focused on their work time, the nutritional value of their food, and the quantities produced. Such studies demonstrate that most of these peoples lead a comfortable life. Geographical environments that we believe to be disadvantaged, given our ignorance of their natural resources, conceal for those who live there a profusion of plant species quite suitable for nourishment. The Indians in the desert regions of California, where a small white population has a difficult time subsisting, were familiar with and consumed dozens of wild plants of great nutritional value. In South Africa it was observed that, even during years of severe drought, millions of nuts of the genus *Ricinodendron*—from which the Bushmen draw part of their nourishment—were rotting on the ground. Once their alimentary needs were met, no one bothered anymore to gather up the nuts.

It has been calculated that, among groups living primarily from hunting or from the gathering of wild products, one man provided for the needs of four or five people. That is, his productivity rate was higher than that of many European peasants on the eve of World War II. This was all the more true in that the time devoted to searching for food was no more than two or three hours a day on average, for a yield exceeding two thousand calories per person (an average that includes children and the elderly) of a very well-balanced diet. One Indian tribe in the Amazonian forest consumes daily more than twice the protein and calories required by international standards, and six times the vitamin C! If the time devoted to cooking the food and manufacturing the implements is added, several populations in America, Africa, and Australia have a work time that does not surpass four hours a day. In actuality, every active adult works six hours a day but only two and a half days a week. The rest of the time is spent on social and religious activity, rest, and leisure.

Nothing obliges us to think that these conditions of existence provide a picture of those that humanity as a whole experienced just prior to the dawn of the Neolithic period. Apart from Australians and a few others, most hunter-gatherers observed by contemporary ethnologists may be the product of a regressive evolution. They were also not immune to hard times. Granted, they knew how to keep the size of their population in equilibrium with the natural environment, thanks to their rules concerning marriage and their various other prohibitions, which limited demographic density to about one person per two square kilometers. It does not follow that all individuals drew an equal benefit from these measures.

In any event, these living conditions explain, at least in part, why these groups did not need or wish to cultivate land and raise livestock, even though preagricultural techniques were perfectly well known to them.

Peoples without agriculture know to burn fields of wild plants at the end of the season, to ensure a better harvest the next year. Near their houses they put in gardens of favorite foods, composed of transplanted specimens. They create original habitats for these species, such as garbage heaps, trails, and burned fields. Many plants that will later be cultivated have an affinity for disturbed soil of that kind and thereby acquire desirable morphological traits: gigantism, well-developed comestible parts, early maturation. These peoples also unintentionally propagate food plants by dropping part of their harvest on the ground. They know the plants, and they know how to help them survive.

The Australian aborigines, who lived without agriculture, were nevertheless metaphorical farmers, so to speak: they observed complicated rites to protect wild plants, to encourage them to grow and multiply, and to keep away parasites and natural disasters. Perhaps we ought to see a certain myth—of which many examples are known throughout the world—as a first image, it too metaphorical, of the domestication of animals. Its hero is endowed with supernatural powers. He pens up wild animals in an enclosure or cave, lets them out only one at a time to provide for his family, or keeps them all so as to cause famine. Fifteen or twenty thousand years ago, Magdalenian hunters may have been breeding livestock symbolically when, in the limited space of caves, they gathered together diverse figurations of animals to decorate the walls.

In short, all the mental faculties and most of the technologies required for agriculture and the domestication of animals existed in germ before these activities appeared. They cannot be considered the result of sudden discoveries. If hunter-gatherers do not cultivate the land, even though they would be perfectly capable of doing so, it is because—rightly or wrongly—they believe they live better without agriculture. Usually, in fact, they know of the farming way of life practiced by neighboring populations. But they refuse to imitate their neighbors because in their view cultivating the land requires too much work and leaves too little leisure time. And that is something that investigations in the field have abundantly confirmed: farming, even when practiced in a rudimentary manner, is harder and takes up more time than hunting and gathering, and it yields less.

Hence the problem raised by historians and ethnologists: If agriculture was neither necessary nor desirable, why did it appear? They have argued passionately about the matter for some thirty years, and it appears that what were formerly seen as consequences of the agricultural revolution are now perceived as its causes: demographic pressure, sedentism, the diversification of the social structure.

There were sedentary peoples who did not practice agriculture. The most famous examples were the fishermen of the Jōmon period in eastern Japan, several millennia BCE; and, until the early nineteenth century, the Indians of the Pacific Coast of Canada, who also lived by fishing, resided in large villages, and had a complicated social organization. It also seems that, in a few places in the Near East, life in permanent villages preceded agricultural economies.

An appealing theory has it that agriculture originated when small groups of people, displaced to a habitat different from their own, were compelled to maintain, despite unfavorable conditions, the preagricultural techniques they had already been practicing elsewhere. We would thus find on the order of culture the conditions that the punctualist biologists postulate to explain the appearance of new natural species. It has also been noted that originally, and for a very long time afterward, agriculture appears to have been limited to incidental products intended to supplement certain seasonal gaps in hunting and gathering.

But there is agreement that, when considered from a more general perspective, neither agriculture nor the domestication of animals was developed to satisfy purely economic needs. Domestic animals were a luxury, a sign of wealth, a symbol of prestige—as can still be observed in India and Africa—well before they were seen as a source of food or raw materials. In the Near East, the domestication of sheep dates back about eleven thousand years, but it was only five thousand years later that use was first made of their wool. In the Americas and in Southeast Asia, the first plants were cultivated less for their nutritional value than as luxury products: condiments, industrial crops, and rare species, isolated specimens of which were identified and protected. That was the case for chili peppers and sisals in Mexico; for cotton and calabashes in South America; for sunflowers, lamb's quarters, and elderberries in the eastern part of North America; for betel or areca nuts in Thailand. Human beings set out to increase the number of rare plants rather than to propagate food plants that were abundant enough in their wild state to satisfy their needs.

The Indian tribes of California traded with one another to obtain not ordinary products for consumption but luxury items: minerals, obsidian, feathers, round shells, and so on. It is remarkable, in fact, that the technological discoveries that made possible the great arts of civilization, such as pottery and metallurgy, were at first used only to produce ornaments and jewelry. The most ancient chemical compound produced by industrial means may have been tetracalcium phosphate, a process entailing several stages. But it was not produced for economic reasons: about seventeen thousand years ago, the Magdalenian painters invented the process to obtain a pigment of a particular shade. They were motivated by aesthetic concerns.

We should not attempt to reduce all types of social development to a single model; rather, we should acknowledge that human societies have conceived of their productive activities in different ways. Hunter-gatherers and farmers do not represent different stages in an evolution obligatory for all. From several standpoints, agriculture was progress: it produces more food in a given space and time and allows for more rapid population growth, a denser occupation of land, and more extensive social groups. But seen from a different perspective, agriculture represented a regression. The human diet deteriorated as a result. It was henceforth limited to a few products rich in calories but poor in nutrients: of the some thousand plants known to be or to have been alimentary resources, agriculture retained only about twenty. And that is not all. In restricting its range of products, farming risks turning a bad harvest into a disaster. It also requires more labor. It may even be that, along with the domestication of animals, it was responsible for the spread of infectious diseases, as suggested by the coincidence in Africa, in both time and space, of the diffusion of agriculture and of sickle-cell anemia, the gene for which, if inherited from only one parent, offers protection against malaria, which progressed in tandem with the clearing of land.

Such phenomena do not belong to the past alone. In response to World War II, Argentina increased its cultivation of corn in order to export it to Europe. As a result, field mice proliferated, and with them cases of viral hemorrhagic fever, since the rodents are carriers of the disease. Other viruses spread by agricultural operations are now rampant in Bolivia, Brazil, China, and Japan. Indeed, carriers of infectious diseases thrive in ecological sites created by humans, such as garbage heaps, cleared land, stagnant pools of water, and so on.

In large modern societies, doing without agriculture is a luxury we can no longer afford: we have tens or hundreds of millions of mouths to feed. If our ancestors had dispensed with farming, as they still could have done, humanity's evolution would have been different. When compared to the size of our population, that of hunter-gatherers appears derisory. But can we claim that the fantastic growth of the population over the entire expanse of the earth has represented progress? All the diverse forms of productive activity over the millennia constitute choices. Each offers advantages, but we must pay the price, consenting to endure the damaging effects.

3

SOCIAL PROBLEMS

RITUAL FEMALE EXCISION AND MEDICALLY ASSISTED REPRODUCTION

In the last few decades, the relationship between ethnologists and the people they study has changed profoundly. Formerly colonized countries, now independent, reproach ethnologists for slowing economic development by encouraging the survival of old practices and outdated beliefs. For nations that are eager to modernize, ethnology looks like the last incarnation of colonialism, and they display mistrust if not hostility toward it.

Elsewhere, the indigenous minorities who survive within a few large modern states—Canada, the United States, Australia, Brazil—have become acutely aware of their ethnic identity and their moral and legal rights. These small communities now refuse to be treated as objects of study by ethnologists, whom they see as parasites and even intellectual exploiters. With the expansion of industrial civilization, the number of societies that have preserved a traditional way of life and can still serve as fodder for ethnologists has greatly diminished. At the same time, the vogue for the social and human sciences in the wake of World War II multiplied the number of researchers. Even fifty years ago, people joked within the profession that an Indian family in the United States had at least three members: the husband, the wife, and the ethnologist. The situation has only gotten worse since then, and indigenous groups, exasperated at being the prey of ethnologists, are rebelling. Some demand that all kinds of forms be filled out to their satisfaction before you are allowed to enter their preserve. Others quite simply prohibit ethnological research: you can come to them as a teacher or health worker, provided you pledge in writing that you will ask no questions about their social organization or religious beliefs. In a pinch, an informant will recount a myth, but only in return for a formal contract acknowledging that it is his or her intellectual property.

In a curious twist, however, the old relationship between the ethnologist and the peoples he studies, rather than being severed, is reversed. Tribes appeal to ethnologists and even hire them to assist them in court, whether to help them assert their ancestral rights over lands or to have the treaties formerly imposed on them voided. This is happening in Australia, where aborigines—and the ethnologists in their service—have attempted several times to prevent the government from installing rocket launch sites or from granting mining concessions in territories held to be sacred. Under similar conditions in Canada and the United States, courts have heard and continue to hear cases concerning the possession of sometimes enormous areas of land. The Indians of Brazil are beginning to organize nationally, and initiatives of the same kind may well be taken there. In such instances, the ethnologist's work completely changes in nature. Once he used the indigenous peoples; now it is they who use him. Adventure, with its aura of poetry and lyricism, is giving way to austere research in libraries, the laborious analysis of the archives to support the case being made and to find legal remedies. Bureaucracy and procedure supplant picturesque "fieldwork," or at the very least transform its spirit.

*
* *

French ethnologists did not expect to have that sort of experience in their own country. Yet that is what is happening, because of the scope that immigration, especially from sub-Saharan Africa, has assumed. For the last year or two, lawyers have been turning to ethnologists for assistance in defending African immigrants who have performed ritual excision on their female children or have had it performed by professionals. Feminist organizations and others dedicated to the protection of children have appeared as witnesses for the prosecution in the legal proceedings initiated by the state. In French law, ritual excision, initially defined as a simple offense falling under the jurisdiction of the criminal courts, became in 1988 a felony tried in the assize court, equated with willful assault and battery against the person of the child leading to mutilation, for which the parents may be found guilty.

A case of this kind tried in 1988 caused a stir because the child had died—not, it seems, from the ritual excision itself but from complications that went untreated. The charge of neglect, or of failure to provide assistance to a person in danger, was thus added to that of assault and battery. In early October 1989 the assize court of Paris heard another case of ritual excision, in which the procedure had had no harmful consequences for the child. But the punishment imposed in both cases was exactly the same: a three-year suspended sentence. Nothing better illustrates the awkward situation in which the courts find themselves. Whatever the outcome of the procedure, fatal or benign, they feel obliged both to condemn and to pardon.

Female ritual excision, commonly practiced by various peoples of Africa and Indonesia (and already in ancient Egypt), consists of the ablation of the clitoris and sometimes also of the labia minora. A girl on whom the procedure is not performed would be considered impure, even dangerous, and would not find a husband. Despite what Europeans often imagine, the practice is not imposed by men; it is "the women's secret," as the interpreters for the accused explained in the 1988 trial. Women want their daughters to have the procedure just as they themselves did.

In initiating legal proceedings, the public prosecutor's office is acting under pressure from public opinion, over which feminist leagues and other well-intentioned organizations exercise a monopoly. How do they justify their indignation?

The first and foremost grievance, it seems, is that ritual excision supposedly eliminates female sexual pleasure, which our societies have made a new article in the declaration of human rights. Second grievance: excision is said to constitute an attack on the integrity of the child's body.

It is surprising that the second argument has never been invoked against male circumcision, which, however, constitutes an assault of the same kind. Some will point out that male circumcision is a benign procedure with none of the major disadvantages that are imputed to female excision. But is that true? I had an excellent friend from an old Breton Catholic family; he was convinced that circumcision reduced the quality of male pleasure, and he would not back down. In the case of female excision, opinions differ. So imprecise is our knowledge of the indirect role of the erogenous zones that we would do better to admit that we know nothing about it. At the October 1989 trial, an African medical doctor who had been excised declared that she had never felt shortchanged in that respect. She added that it was not until she came to Paris that she learned that excised women were frigid.

In any case, it is clear that, even without any consequences for male pleasure, circumcision constitutes an attack on the physical integrity of the boy's body, a violent trace that, like female excision, obliges him to perceive himself as different from other children. It is therefore not clear why the argument invoked in the second case is not also used in the first—unless it is because our Judeo-Christian culture is still steeped in the Old Testament and that such familiarity removes any shocking aspect male circumcision might have. Circumcision (for the Jews directly and for the Christians indirectly) belongs to a shared cultural heritage. It is for that reason and that reason alone that it does not disturb us.

Lawyers called upon to provide a defense in trials for ritual excision have solicited ethnologists' opinion in an effort to choose between two defenses. They are tempted to plead lack of responsibility because they are persuaded—and think they can persuade the judges—that in societies defined as backward, individuals do not have free will but are rather totally subject to the constraints exerted by the group. Such individuals therefore cannot be held responsible for their actions. Ethnologists do not follow jurists down that path. They know that that way of envisioning societies wrongly called primitive or archaic is one of the outdated ideas of nineteenth-century thought. In all societies there is a great variety of individual behaviors. Members adhere more or less faithfully to the norms of the group; strictly speaking, no one is incapable of deviating from them. By means of that defense, lawyers might obtain leniency for their clients, but in the process they would discredit them and their culture. Paradoxically, defense attorneys would be shoring up the clear conscience of the prosecutors since they would agree to acknowledge the absolute superiority of the civilization on whose behalf the legal proceedings were initiated and in the name of which the court will pronounce its verdict.

Ethnologists will instead try to make the judges understand how beliefs that we ourselves judge barbaric or ridiculous are warranted for those who adhere to them. Everywhere in the world where female excision or male circumcision is practiced (and often these practices occur in tandem), the underlying logic seems to be the same: the Creator, in establishing the distinction between the sexes, did not perform his job properly. Whether because he was in too much of a hurry, careless, or distracted in his work, he left a trace of masculinity in women, a trace of femininity in men. The ablation of the clitoris or the foreskin has the result of completing that work, ridding each sex of a residual impurity and making each conform to its respective nature. That metaphysics and that way of thinking are alien to us. Nevertheless, we can recognize their coherence and not be impervious to their beauty and grandeur.

Instead of relegating the accused to some subhuman state, thereby unwittingly validating racial prejudices, we should endeavor to show that practices that are meaningless within one cultural order may be meaningful in another. Indeed, there is no common measure by which to judge systems of beliefs or, a fortiori, to condemn one or another of them, unless we claim—but on what basis?—that only one (ours, of course) conveys universal values and must be imposed on all.

There are no grounds for punishing, in the name of a particular moral code, people who are simply following practices dictated by a different code. Does that mean we must tolerate them? The conclusion is not self-evident. The ethnologist and the moralist make an objective observation: in our country, ritual female excision is an affront to the public conscience. Our system of values, which has as much right to respect as any other, would be profoundly weakened if, on the same soil, customs felt to be incompatible could freely coexist. Ritual excision trials thus have an exemplary value. The idea that one might condemn the defendants is absurd. But an ethical choice, with the future of the host country's culture hanging in the balance, can be made only between two possibilities: either proclaim that anything that can be justified on the basis of custom is permitted everywhere; or send back to their own country those who—as is their right—intend to remain faithful to their practices even if, on whatever grounds, they gravely offend the sensitivities of their hosts. The only excuse to be found for the decisions of 1988 and 1989 is that, in the eyes of the accused, a conviction with a suspended sentence probably represented a milder punishment than expulsion from the country.

*
* *

In another realm as well, ethnologists are being thrust onto the public stage. Some have been invited to sit on commissions that were formed to give an opinion to the governments of various countries on the new methods of medically assisted reproduction. Faced with the advances in the life sciences, public opinion vacillates. Several methods for producing a child are available to infertile couples: artificial insemination, egg donation, the use of surrogate mothers for hire or free of cost, in vitro fertilization with sperm provided by the husband or by another man and with an egg from the wife or another woman. Is everything to be allowed? Should certain procedures be permitted and others banned? And if so, on what basis?

Previously unknown legal situations arise for which the laws of European countries do not have a ready answer. In contemporary societies, the idea that filiation is the result of a biological connection tends to prevail over the idea that it is a social bond. In English law, social paternity does not even exist: the sperm donor could legally claim the child or be obliged to support it. In France the Napoleonic Code stipulates that the mother's husband is the child's legal father. It therefore rejects biological paternity in favor of social paternity: *Pater id est quem nuptiae demonstrant.* Nevertheless, a 1972 law belies that old adage by allowing paternity suits to go forward. We therefore no longer know whether the social or the biological relationship takes precedence. What responses, then, are we to give to the problems raised by medically assisted reproduction in cases where the child's legal father is not the biological father and where the mother has not herself provided the egg or perhaps the uterus in which gestation takes place?

Depending on the case, a child born of such procedures may have one father and one mother as usual, or one mother and two fathers, two mothers and one father, two mothers and two fathers, three mothers and one father, or even three mothers and two fathers, if the sperm donor is not the father and if three women participate: the one donating an egg, the one providing her uterus, and the one who will be the child's legal mother.

What will the respective rights and duties of the social and the biological parents be, now that they are different people? How should a court decide in a case where the surrogate mother delivers a disabled child, and the couple that employed her services rejects it? Or conversely, if a woman inseminated by the husband of an infertile woman and on her behalf changes her mind and decides to keep the child as her own? Must all desires be considered legitimate? That of a woman who asks to be inseminated with the frozen sperm of her deceased husband? That of two lesbians who want to have a child with an egg from one of them artificially fertilized by an anonymous donor and implanted in the other's uterus?

Can surrogacy or sperm or egg donation be the object of a contract requiring payment? Must they be anonymous, or may the social parents and eventually the child itself know the identity of the biological parents? None of these questions is gratuitous: these problems and others even more outlandish have been and continue to be raised in court. All this appears so new that judges, lawmakers, and even moralists, lacking experience with comparable situations, find themselves at a complete loss.

Not so ethnologists, the only ones who were not caught off guard by this sort of problem. Granted, the societies they study are unacquainted with the modern techniques of in vitro fertilization, the removal of an egg or embryo, its transfer and implantation into a uterus, and the freezing of sperm, eggs, and embryos. But they have imagined metaphorical equivalents. And since they believe in the reality of these metaphors, the psychological and legal implications are the same.

My colleague Françoise Héritier-Augé has shown that insemination with donor sperm has an equivalent in Africa, among the Samo of Burkina Faso. Girls in that society are married off very young, and each must take an official lover for a certain period of time before going to live with her husband. When the moment comes, she brings her husband the child she has had by her lover; that child will be considered the firstborn of the legitimate union. A man may take several wives; if they leave him he remains the legal father of all the children they later bear.

In other African populations as well, a husband who has been abandoned by one or more of his wives has a right of paternity over future children. He need only have the first postpartum sexual relations with his former wife after she has become a mother. That act determines who will be the legal father of the next child. A man married to an infertile woman may thus arrange for a fertile woman to name him the father, gratis or in exchange for payment. In that case, the woman's husband is the sperm donor, and the woman leases her uterus to another man or a childless couple. The burning question in France as to whether the surrogate mother must provide her services without charge or whether she may receive remuneration therefore does not arise in Africa.

The Nuer of Sudan consider an infertile woman the equivalent of a man; she can therefore marry a woman. Among the Yoruba of Nigeria, rich women buy wives for themselves, sending them off to live with men. When a child is born, the woman who is the legal "husband" claims it or cedes it to the biological father in exchange for payment. In the first case, a couple composed of two women, who can therefore be defined as homosexual in the literal sense of the word, practice assisted reproduction in order to have children; one of the women will be the legal father, the other the biological mother.

The institution of the levirate, in force among the ancient Hebrews and still widespread throughout the world, allows and at time even requires that a younger brother sire a child in the name of his dead brother. This is the equivalent of insemination postmortem. An even clearer case is the "ghost marriage" of the Nuer of Sudan: if a man died a bachelor or without offspring, a close relative could take enough of the deceased's livestock to purchase a wife. He would then produce a son (whom he considered his nephew) in the name of the deceased. Sometimes that son would in turn perform the same function vis-à-vis his biological father—legally, his uncle. The children he produced would therefore legally be his cousins.

In all these examples, the child's social status is determined by the legal father, even if that father is a woman. Nevertheless, the child knows the identity of its biological father; the two are united by bonds of affection. Contrary to our fears, transparency does not cause the child to feel any conflict about the fact that its biological father and its social father are two different individuals.

There are societies in Tibet where several brothers share a wife. All the offspring are attributed to the eldest, whom the children call "father." They call the other men their uncles. The real biological connections are not unknown, but they are granted little importance. A symmetrical situation prevailed in the Amazon rainforest among the Tupi-Kawahib, whom I knew fifty years ago. A man could marry several sisters or a mother and her daughter from a previous union; these women reared their children together, showing little concern, it seemed, about whether the child a woman was caring for was her own or that of another of her husband's wives.

The conflict between biological kinship and social kinship, which in Europe troubles jurists and moralists, does not exist, therefore, in the societies known to ethnologists. These societies give primacy to the social, but the two aspects do not clash in the group's ideology or in its members' consciousness. It should not be concluded that our society ought to model its conduct on such exotic examples. But these examples can at least accustom us to the idea that the problems raised by medically assisted reproduction allow for a good number of different solutions, none of which should be considered natural and self-evident.

In fact, we need not look so far off to be convinced. In matters of assisted reproduction, one of our major concerns seems to be to separate fertilization from sexuality and even, as it were, from sensuality. To be acceptable, everything must take place in the sanitized atmosphere of the laboratory, anonymously and through the intervention of the physician, in such a way as to exclude any personal contact, any sharing of eroticism or emotion between the participants. Before the advent of modern technologies, however, sperm donation was not unknown in our societies, but that type of service was rendered without a fuss and, as it were, "close to home." In 1843, at a time when social and moral prejudices were much stronger than they are today, Balzac began a novel he never finished and which he called, significantly, "The Petty Bourgeois." This novel, undoubtedly inspired by real events, tells of an agreement between two couples, one fertile, the other infertile, who are friends: the fertile woman takes on the task of producing a child with the infertile woman's husband. The daughter born of that union is pampered in equal measure by the two couples, who live in the same building, and everyone around them knows of the situation.

In answer to jurists and moralists impatient to make laws, the ethnologist therefore dispenses this piece of advice: Be cautious. He points out that even practices and demands most shocking to public opinion—medically assisted reproduction for unmarried women, single men, widows, or homosexual couples—have their equivalents in other societies, which are none the worse for it.

The wise course, no doubt, is to trust that the internal logic of every society's institutions and system of values will create viable family structures and will eliminate those that produce contradictions. Only time will tell what will be accepted or rejected in the long run by the collective consciousness.

*
* *

Ethnologists often hear it said that their discipline is doomed because of the rapid extinction of the traditional cultures that formed its field of study. In a standardized world where every group aspires to the same cultural model, what place remains for differences? The two examples I have given, that of ritual female excision and that of medically assisted reproduction, show that the problems raised for the ethnologist by the world as it now exists are not disappearing: they are simply shifting. Female excision did not trouble the Western conscience when it was practiced far away, in exotic countries with which there was little contact. Even in the eighteenth century, authors such as Buffon wrote of it with indifference. If we now feel it is of concern to us, it is because the mobility of populations, and especially the scope that immigration from Africa has taken on, brings ritual incision home to us, as it were. Incompatible customs, which were able to coexist peacefully at a distance, collide when suddenly brought into proximity with each other. And if medically assisted reproduction also creates problems of conscience, it is for the opposite but symmetrical reason: a gap is opening within our own society between traditional morality and the advances of science. Here again, we do not know whether or how it is possible to reconcile situations that appear contradictory. The fact that in both cases people turn to ethnologists, call them in for consultations, urge them to give their views (which, in fact, are not followed), clearly shows that ethnologists still have a function to perform. The advent of a global civilization makes the clash between external differences sharper, and it does not prevent internal differences from erupting within a particular society. Ethnologists, as the saying goes, still have a lot on their plate.

4

PRESENTATION OF A BOOK

BY ITS AUTHOR

Histoire de Lynx (Paris: Plon, 1991; *The Story of Lynx*), written in old age, will probably be my last book—the last, in any case, that I intend to devote to Native American mythology. It was published toward the end of this year, 1991, on the eve of the five hundredth anniversary of the discovery of the New World. It was therefore natural that the book should take the form of a tribute to Amerindians: ever since I first encountered them in 1935, their customs, their social institutions, their religious beliefs, their philosophical thought, and their arts have provided me with food for thought.

This choice was not at all premeditated, however. It imposed itself as I was writing my book: at first I set out simply to solve a specific problem, so specific that, having run into it several times, I had excluded it from my previous books, promising myself that, God willing, I would return to it one day.

Myths from the Pacific Northwest of the United States and Canada establish parallels and oppositions between the origin of fog and that of wind: parallels in that these myths belong to a single totality; and oppositions in that, whereas fog is attributed a true origin, wind is already in existence when the mythic narrative begins. Wind appears in the guise of a man with a very big head topping a body so thin and light that it flutters back and forth without touching the ground, or as a round, hollow, and boneless body that bounces like a ball. That evil creature persecutes human beings. A young Indian manages to capture it and then free it, but only in exchange for a promise: the wind will henceforth blow with moderation. Fog, which interposes itself between heaven and earth, is what can be called a spatial mediator; wind, by contrast, which pledges to become intermittent and to follow the rhythm of the seasons, is a temporal mediator.

All the myths relating to these two meteorological phenomena are part of a vast system where the same incidents and the same actors recur. The myths are nested one inside the other like Russian dolls. Those about capturing the wind, which have the richest plot, are situated on the periphery; those about the origin of fog, often barely sketched out, occupy the center. I therefore found it useful to begin with them.

At first sight, these myths appear to be little tales without any cosmological implications. At a time when humans and animals did not yet form distinct categories, a sick and repulsive old man named Lynx, whether intentionally or accidentally, impregnated the daughter of a chief by letting a trickle of saliva or urine run over her—or sometimes by other procedures. The child was born. An ordeal was arranged to find out which of all the men in the village was its father. The baby pointed to Lynx. Then the indignant villagers beat him almost to death and abandoned him, along with his wife and son. Lynx was transformed into a beautiful and vigorous young man, a great hunter who provided lavishly for his little family. But he sent a thick fog over the new village where his persecutors had settled; that fog made hunting impossible and caused a famine. The residents asked for forgiveness and received it. Lynx became the chief of the village.

This story, of no great import apart from its moral, is found in the same form or in very similar forms from one end of the Americas to the other. In the years that immediately followed the discovery of the New World, it was heard by travelers and missionaries in Mexico, Brazil, and Peru. Despite its apparent insignificance, it displays an astonishing stability, not only across space—from Canada to the banks of the South Atlantic to the Andes—but also across time, since narratives collected more than four centuries ago differ little from those that can be heard today.

In the Canadian versions of this myth—a kernel of those on the origin of fog, which was born from the old, unhealthy skin that the hero sheds—Lynx's principal enemy is Coyote, who also plays an important role in the other series of myths, the one about the wind's capture. Lynx is a Felidae, Coyote a Canidae. There is nothing surprising about the marked opposition between the two families: Do we not say of two people who do not get along that they fight like cats and dogs? In the early nineteenth century, a very minor poet named Marc-Antoine Désaugiers composed a ditty in which each verse contrasted "like dog and cat" not only Voltaire and Rousseau, Grétry and Rossini, the classic and the romantic, but also duty and pleasure, morality and desire, justice and fairness. No doubt the philosophical import given to the opposition was simply a pleasantry in his view, as it remains in ours. But in their myths the Amerindians confer on it a fullness of meaning and draw all the requisite consequences.

According to them, the opposition did not exist in the beginning. Once upon a time, they say, Lynx and Coyote were close friends and had the same morphology. But they quarreled, and in revenge Lynx lengthened Coyote's muzzle, paws, and tail; Coyote pushed in Lynx's muzzle and shortened his tail. Since that time, they have had contrasting physical appearances: one is extroverted, the other introverted.

Both physically and morally, then, Lynx and Coyote, the Felidae and the Canidae, may have been and might have remained something like twins. The myths suggest, however, that this would have been contrary to the order of the world, which required that two beings, similar at first, should become different. The importance that the myths grant to these little stories is therefore clear. Figuratively, they introduce the notion of an impossible twinship, which holds a central place in the Amerindians' philosophical thought.

In fact, Amerindians conceive of the genesis of beings and things in terms of a series of bipartitions. In the beginning the demiurge separated himself from his creatures, who were subdivided into Indians and non-Indians. Then the Indians themselves split into two groups, countrymen and enemies. A new distinction appeared among countrymen, between the good and the wicked; and the good were in turn divided between the strong and the weak. At several places along that sequence of dichotomies, brothers intervened: twins or nearly so (sometimes they had different fathers), they had disparate talents and were the agents of one or another of the divisions. One was peaceful, the other bellicose; one wise, the other foolish; one deft, the other clumsy; and so on. Indeed, no true equality may appear between the resulting parts at any stage: in some way, one is always superior to the other.

What these myths implicitly proclaim is that the oppositions that organize natural phenomena and life in society—heaven and earth, up and down, fire and water, fog and wind, near and far, Indians and non-Indians, countrymen and strangers, and so on—will never be symmetrical, even though each term of the pair implies the other. The mind strives to pair them up, but without managing to establish parity between them. The same always engenders the other. The smooth operation of the universe depends on that dynamic imbalance; otherwise, at every moment the universe would run the risk of falling into a state of inertia.

That explains why twinship, which occupies such a large place in the mythology of the Amerindians, never appears in its pure state. It would be surprising were that not the case, since, at least in the South American tropics but often elsewhere as well, Indians feared the birth of twins and put one or both of them to death. In myths, divine or heroic twins can play a positive role, because their twinship remains incomplete and is related to the particular circumstances of their conception or birth. That is also the case for Castor and Pollux:

but the Dioscuri strove to become the same and succeeded in doing so, whereas in the Americas twins never overcome the initial rift that existed between them. They even apply themselves to widening it, as if a metaphysical necessity constrained all originally paired terms to diverge. A set of consequences follows: at the cosmological level, the impossibility of reconciling extremes, which, despite a wistful dream, will never be able to be twins; and, at the sociological and economic level, a perpetual seesawing back and forth, between war and commerce with the outside world, between reciprocity and hierarchy within the society.

Of all these bipartitions, it is primarily that between whites and Indians that holds our attention. The first Brazilian myth known in Europe was the great myth of the origin of the Tupinamba, collected by the French Cordeliers monk André Thevet in about 1550–55 and published in his *Cosmographie universelle* (*Universal Cosmography*; 1575). In it we read that in the early days of the world, the demiurge lived among his creatures and showered his blessings on them. But the creatures proved to be ungrateful, and the demiurge destroyed them. He saved one man, however, and created a woman so that they could reproduce. Thus was born a new race and, above all, the second demiurge, master of all the arts. Whites are the true children of that demiurge, since their culture surpasses that of the Indians.

The distinction between whites and Indians thus made its appearance in the early days of creation. As Alfred Métraux has already noted, myths of the same kind arose in many Indian tribes, too soon after the conquest for these resemblances to be explained away as borrowings. If the profound structure of the Amerindian myths is truly what I have set it out to be, the difficulty disappears.

These myths, as I said, proceed by introducing successive rifts between beings and things. The two parts, ideally twins at every stage, always prove to be unequal. And no imbalance could appear greater to the Indians than that between them and the whites. Yet they possessed a binary model, prefabricated as it were, that allowed them to transpose en bloc the opposition and its consequences into a system where a place was seemingly set aside for it. Hence, as soon as the opposition was introduced, it began to function. The Indians' system accounted for the existence of the other as a metaphysical presupposition.

The historical evidence provides confirmation for this interpretation. From one end of the New World to the other, Indians proved to be extraordinarily well disposed toward welcoming the whites, making a place for them, providing them with everything they desired and more. That was the treatment—which was not repaid in kind, far from it—that Columbus received in the Bahamas and the West Indies, Cortés in Mexico, Pizarro in Peru, Cabral and Villegaignon in Brazil, and Cartier in Canada. But that is because, well before the arrival of the whites, in Amerindian thinking the very existence of the Indians implied that of non-Indians. Both in Mexico and in the Andes, the traditions collected in the wake of the conquest attest that the Amerindians were in fact expecting the whites. That enigmatic prescience can therefore be explained.

In the Pacific Northwest of the United States and Canada, encounters with whites occurred at a later date. Not until the eighteenth century did the Indians have contact with Spanish, English, French, and Russian sailors. Once the fur trade got under way in the nineteenth century, it was primarily with French Canadians—"voyageurs," they were called at the time—that contacts multiplied. The welcoming disposition I have indicated as characteristic of Amerindians was demonstrated within a narrower framework, but it is still of great interest for the study of myths. Indian traditions were very receptive to those of the new arrivals, and the myths of the region are so profoundly pervaded by popular French tales that it is sometimes difficult to distinguish between autochthonous elements and borrowings.

The mental attitude of the Indians, as manifested in philosophical thought and in the creation of narratives, contrasts strikingly with that of Europeans vis-à-vis the peoples of the New World. In the first decades after the discovery of America, they displayed indifference toward both people and things from that part of the world, an intentional blindness in the face of too many novelties, which Europeans refused to recognize as such. For those living in the sixteenth century, that discovery did not so much reveal the diversity of customs as demonstrate it. The discovery of the New World was dwarfed by others: that of Egyptian, Greek, and Roman mores, which the great authors of antiquity had already made known. The spectacle of the peoples recently discovered only provided confirmation for those earlier accounts. If not déjà vu, it was all at least *déjà su*, already known. That withdrawal into oneself, that skittishness, that willful blindness were the response of a group that, having believed it constituted humankind as a whole, suddenly discovered that it was only half the human race.

In the case of Montaigne, who came along a little later, the knowledge of Amerindian customs, which he drew from travel narratives, no doubt provided in part the foundations for a critique of our own institutions and mores. But Montaigne's radical skepticism led to the conclusion that, if all institutions are equally valid, and as such open to criticism and respectable in equal measure, wisdom advises us to embrace those of the society in which we live. In practice if not in theory, that line of conduct did not diverge from that of the missionaries of the period and of subsequent centuries, who saw the Catholic faith as the sole rampart against bewildering customs and beliefs irreconcilable with their own.

Histoire de Lynx is the seventh book (along with many articles) that I will have devoted to Amerindian mythology. Following on the four volumes of *Mythologiques* (translated into English as *Introduction to the Study of Mythology*), it forms a trilogy with *La voie des masques* (*The Way of the Masks*) and *La potière jalouse* (*The Jealous Potter*). In all these books I attempted to give a vast body of oral literature its rightful place. This literature is too little known, having remained buried in often largely inaccessible scholarly collections. In terms of its grandeur, its interest, and its beauties, it is in no way inferior to the traditions bequeathed to us by classical antiquity, the Celtic world, and Eastern and Far Eastern civilizations. This literature too belongs to humanity's cultural heritage. And if I was able to discover in the "matter of America" (in the sense one speaks of the "matter of Britain," referring to the Grail cycle) a privileged field for shedding new light on the operations of mythic thought, in doing so I merely paid another tribute to the genius of the Amerindians.

The reflections on the encounter between two worlds with which *Histoire de Lynx* ends may allow us to go further, or rather, to return to the philosophical and ethical sources of Amerindian dualism. Georges Dumézil has shown that, in the religious practices and myths of the Indo-Europeans, a tripartite ideology was at work. It seems to me that a different ideology, one that is bipartite, is at work in the beliefs and institutions of Amerindians. But that dualism is not at all static. However it manifests itself, its terms are always in an unstable balance. It thus draws its dynamism from an openness to the other, which found expression in the Indians' welcoming attitude toward the whites, who, however, were motivated by much less friendly dispositions.

As we prepare to celebrate the five-hundredth anniversary of what I would call the invasion of the New World rather than its discovery, the acknowledgment of the brutal destruction of its peoples and of their values will serve as an act of contrition and piety.

5

THE ETHNOLOGIST'S JEWELS

As the frontispiece for his book *On Growth and Form*, which I consider one of the intellectual monuments of our time, D'Arcy Wentworth Thompson chose a picture in extreme close-up, taken at 1/50,000th of a second, depicting a drop of milk falling into the same liquid.[1] The milk that splashes up forms a pattern of remarkable beauty. At the point of impact, a perfectly round ruff flares out, then breaks up into fine serrations, each topped by a miniscule bead of milk.

The author was a biologist. Through that image, he wanted to demonstrate that a complicated form from the physical world, with an appearance so fleeting that only time-lapse photography can capture and record it, is altogether similar to the form that marine animals such as Coelenterata—hydras and jellyfish, for example—gradually assume over the course of their development. The book abounds in examples of this type. The conclusion to be drawn from these comparisons is that the physical and the biological worlds obey the same morphological laws. These laws translate invariant relationships that can be formulated in mathematical terms.

For the historian and the ethnologist, the frontispiece of Thompson's book inspires comparisons of a different order, encouraging them quite simply to broaden the Scottish biologist's thesis to include products of the human mind. The splash of milk prefigures exactly a man-made object whose design would seem to be completely arbitrary—namely, a crown, and more precisely a count's crown. In the art of heraldry, such a crown takes the form of a circle of flared metal, cut into points at the top, each surmounted by a bead (sixteen, actually, rather than the twenty-four of the splash of milk, but the number of points is probably determined by the viscosity of the liquid). Within the hierarchy of the French nobility, the title of count was below that of duke and that of marquis. All three had what were called "open" crowns, as opposed to the closed royal (or imperial) crown, that is, one that incorporates half-circles that meet at the top. It seems that the closed crown was definitively adopted in France by Francis I, so that he would be the equal in all things to Henry VIII of England and Charles V, who had already chosen that type.

Just as the physical world provides an image of the most simple of the open crowns (the marquis's and the duke's crowns were somewhat more complicated), it is not difficult to find images of the closed crown, at least since instant photography has allowed us to see the different stages of an atomic explosion: first the cloud rises, then it widens and closes. In a no less significant analogy, drawn from the biological world this time, this is often called a "mushroom cloud."

Thus we find that royal or nobiliary crowns, bizarre objects that might be taken for artistic whims corresponding to nothing in nature, anticipated a knowledge of the most fleeting states of matter, which were at the time realities as yet unperceived. Moreover, the hierarchy of heraldic symbols directly reflects the hierarchy that can be established between these states in the physical world: the gaseous state has a higher level of instability than the liquid state. And yet it was not until the late nineteenth century, with the advent of chronophotography, that it was discovered that a liquid splash prefigures a count's crown, a gas explosion a royal or imperial crown. The artisans who designed these crowns and invented their forms, lacking suitable methods of observation, could not have possessed a representation of these physical phenomena that they unwittingly imitated.

A first conclusion: goldsmithery and jewelry making are undoubtedly arts in which the human imagination is believed to enjoy free rein, but even the wildest fantasies are products of the human mind, which is part of the world. Before knowing the world from the outside, the mind contemplates within itself a few of the world's realities, all the while believing it is engaging in pure creativity.

That is not all. These crowns, which depicted unstable states of matter at a time when the fleetingness of these states made them impossible to capture, were covered with precious stones. In an exhibition currently being held in Paris, which assembles what remains of the royal treasures, the coronation crown of Louis XV is on view.[2] In its original state, it was adorned with 282 diamonds, 64 colored gems (16 rubies, 16 sapphires, 16 emeralds, and 16 topazes), and 230 pearls, all of which were replaced by copies in the eighteenth century. On this figuration, still unconscious at the time, of one of the most unstable states of matter—since this is a closed crown—gems were included, as they generally were on royal or nobiliary crowns. Like the metals from which these crowns are made (iron, silver, and gold), these gems constitute the most stable bodies in the physical world, so much so that they can be called imperishable.

Has not the principal aim of the art of jewelry, and not only that of crowns, always been to associate and combine the extreme states that matter is capable of assuming? The jewels that most astonish and captivate us are those that best succeed in uniting solidity and fragility—for example, the light, trembling leaves of gold with which ladies of Ur adorned themselves in the third millennium. It is as if the ideal goal of the gold worker and jeweler were always and everywhere to enchase hard, geometrical, incorruptible stones in a setting of precious metal, which, by the delicacy of its workmanship, evokes the grace, caprice, and precariousness of living forms.

*

* *

Let us consider the problem in broader terms. Human beings in the past could not have imagined the form taken for a fraction of a second by a liquid splash or a gaseous explosion. But an image of instability was immediately available to them: the short duration of an individual's lifespan, given the risks to which one was exposed or, quite simply, natural law. Is not the birth of each creature among a multitude of others and its brief passage on earth similar to tiny splashes or explosions on the surface of the great current of life? In decorating themselves with hard and durable substances that withstand the assaults of time, human beings transposed onto their own bodies the opposition between the stable and the unstable and sought to overcome it. When formulated in anatomical terms, this became the opposition between the hard and the soft, and ethnographic investigations have shown that it occupies the foremost place in the representations of the body by peoples without writing.

The Bororo of central Brazil, with whom I became acquainted more than half a century ago, find in that opposition the principle of their natural philosophy. For them, life connotes activity and hardness, death softening and inertia. They distinguish between two aspects of every corpse, human or animal: first, the soft flesh subject to putrefaction; and second, the incorruptible parts, such as the fangs, claws, and beak for animals; the bones, necklaces, and feather ornaments for humans. One myth tells that the civilizing hero "opened these vile things, the soft parts of the body." He pierced ears, nostrils, and lips so that these parts could be replaced symbolically by hard things, including fingernails, toenails, claws, teeth, fangs, shells, and plant fibers, the very materials used in jewelry, whose significance thus becomes clear. Jewelry turns the soft into the hard; it stands in for the objectionable parts of the body, which prefigure death. Jewels are literally givers of life.

Initially, therefore, it is not very important whether these materials are rare or common: the essential thing is that they be rigid and hard. How many times have I seen an Indian who had lost a nose ring, a pendant earring, or a labret, precious by virtue of its material or workmanship, worry less about finding it than about hurriedly replacing it with some little piece of wood? These objects stand guard in front of bodily orifices, which are the most vulnerable aspects of the soft parts, exposed as they are to penetration by evil beings or influences. It is not without reason that the Aramaic word used in the Bible to designate earrings has the general sense of "holy thing." Other parts of the body, such as the hands and feet, also require protection because they are the most exposed.

The Pacific Coast Indians of Canada used to say of a woman who did not have her ears pierced that she was "earless," and, if she did not wear a labret, that she was "mouthless." The same idea is expressed by certain Indians of Brazil but in more positive terms: according to them, the wood disk they insert in their pierced lower lip gives their words authority; the disks they wear in their earlobes make them capable of understanding and assimilating the words of others.

Such conceptions make distinguishing between jewelry and amulets a pointless exercise. The oldest jewelry known in Europe comes from prehistoric sites dating back thirty or forty thousand years: animal teeth with holes bored into them, so that they could hang from a string. Later came rings or disks of engraved bone, and fragments of carved bones shaped like the heads of horses, bison, or stags. All these objects measured between three and six centimeters and so were apparently too small for any utilitarian function.

It should be remembered that, just a few centuries ago, particular value was attached to diamonds because it was believed they protected against poison; to rubies, because they kept away poisonous vapors; to sapphires, for their sedative properties; to turquoise, which warned of danger; and to amethyst, because it allayed drunkenness, as attested by the meaning of its Greek name, *amethustos*.

In the Old and New Worlds it was obviously gold, once it was discovered, that was seen as the giver of life par excellence. Gold shines like the sun; its physical and chemical properties make it inalterable. When it comes to gold's virtues, unanimity reigns. In the region inhabited by the Bororo, gold was abundant, sometimes lying right on the ground. The word they used for it means approximately "hardened fragment of the sun"; this corresponds closely to the beliefs of the ancient Egyptians, who regarded gold as the sun's brilliant and incorruptible flesh. The poets of classical India sang the praises of gold, the equivalent on earth of the sun in the sky: "Gold is immortal, so too the sun; gold is round because the sun is round. Truly, this golden plaque is the sun." Twenty-five or thirty centuries later, Karl Marx, an occasional poet, would appropriate the comparison, pointing out the aesthetic (and not only economic) qualities of precious metals: "They appear, so to speak, as solidified light raised from a subterranean world, since all the rays of light in their original composition are reflected by silver, while red alone, the colour of the highest potency, is reflected by gold."[3] That transmutation of light, an impalpable element, into a solid metal brings us back to the dialectical opposition between the stable and the unstable with which we began.

In this respect, copper often played a comparable role to that of gold and silver. Gold, found as nuggets or flakes, is immediately recognizable: it is pure and shines in its full splendor when it is picked up. So too copper, which, when found in its native state, also lends itself to hammering. The oldest gold known was mined on the banks of the Black Sea in what is now Bulgaria, in the fifth millennium BCE. And excavations have yielded copper objects as well as gold ones. Also in the fifth millennium, the peoples of pre-Columbian North America, which, with the exception of Mexico, had no gold, fashioned copper objects in large quantities. That predilection for copper persisted among the Pacific Coast Indians of Canada and Alaska until the twentieth century. Their ideas about copper were in all points comparable to those about gold in ancient India and ancient Egypt: it was a solar substance of supernatural origin, a source of life and happiness, the most precious of riches and the symbol of all the others.

Have these beliefs disappeared in our own societies? Certainly not in the case of gold, but one might think so for copper, which is now put to all sorts of common industrial uses. From time to time, however, an advertisement can be seen in French magazines with the following text surrounding the image of a piece of copper jewelry: "Copper, discreet but vital; beautiful, eternal, brilliant, sparkling, universal, warm, rich, unique. Copper makes us more beautiful." The myths of the Pacific Coast Indians are not expressed any differently.

Hence the appeal that jewelry, independent of its value and beauty, has for the ethnologist. It occupies one of those sectors of our culture where what I have called the "savage mind" persists, astonishingly vital. When European women put on earrings, they—and we who look at them—are still dimly aware that they are fortifying the perishable body with imperishable substances. Jewelry, which converts soft parts into hard parts, mediates between life and death. Are not jewels handed down from one generation to the next? They can perform that function only because, when we combine the most stable materials encountered in nature with forms like crowns, which evoke instability, or when we associate their hardness with our own fragility, we all act out in miniature the allegory of an ideal world, where these contradictions would have no occasion to exist.

6

PORTRAITS OF ARTISTS

Among the Plains Indians of North America, the men painted figurative scenes or abstract decorations on bison skins and other objects. For the women, porcupine quill embroidery was the principal mode of artistic expression. The difficult technique took years to master. The quills, which vary in length and strength depending on the part of the animal they come from, first had to be flattened, softened, and dyed. The women then had to learn to bend them, tie them in knots, braid them, interlace them, and sew them. Their sharp tips could cause cruel wounds.

This geometric embroidery, purely decorative in appearance, had a symbolic meaning. It consisted of messages whose form and content the embroiderer had considered at length. She often received them as a revelation: the embroiderer saw in a dream the complicated motif she would have to render; or it appeared to her on a rock or the side of a cliff; or it came to her in its finished form. The supposed originator of the revelation was a two-faced deity, mother of the arts. Once she had inspired a woman to create a new motif, other women copied it, and it became part of the tribal repertoire. But the creator herself remained out of the ordinary.

> "When a woman dreams of the Double Woman," an old informant recounted nearly a century ago, "from that time on, in everything she makes, no one excels her. But then the woman is very much like a crazy woman. . . . She laughs uncontrollably and so time and time again, she acts deceptively. . . . So the people are very afraid of her. She causes all men who stand near her to become possessed. . . . For that reason these women are called Double Women. They are very promiscuous. . . . But then in the things they make nobody excels them. They do much quillwork. From then on, they are very skillful. They also do work like a man."[1]

This astonishing portrait of the artist far outstrips the imagery of romanticism and that of the accursed poet or painter that emerged later in the nineteenth century, with all its pseudo-philosophical variations regarding the relation between art and madness. Where we use figurative expressions, societies without writing speak literally. We have only to transpose their words to recognize that these societies are not so different from our own, or that we are closer to them than we might think.

On the Pacific Coast of western Canada, painters and sculptors belonged to a distinct social category. They were designated by a collective noun that implied they were surrounded by mystery. In fact, any man or woman, or even any child, who caught them at their work was immediately put to death. These were extremely hierarchical societies, and the position of artist was passed on from one generation to the next within the nobility, but commoners whose gifts attracted notice were also admitted. In all cases, aspiring artists were subjected to long and harsh initiation rites. A predecessor had to cast his supernatural power into the body of the one called upon to succeed him, who, ravished by the protective spirit, then vanished into the sky. In reality, he remained hidden in the woods for a variable length of time before reappearing in public, vested with his new powers.

The masks, in fact, which only sculptors had the right and talent to make, were formidable entities. Simple or articulated, they represented different sorts of spirits. According to the account of an educated Indian in the early part of the twentieth century, the mask of a supernatural protector named Boiling Words

> has a body like that of a dog. The chief did not wear it on his face or on his head, because the mask had its own body, and it was considered a very terrible object. Its whistle was very hard to blow. Nobody now knows how to do it. It is not blown with the mouth, but it is squeezed on a certain mark on the whistle. All they knew about this being was that it was living in a rock of the mountain. They had a song of this mask. It was always kept hidden, and no common people knew about it, only the children of the head chief and the children of the head man of Dzēba′sa's tribe. The children were very much afraid to hear the voice of Boiling Words. It was a very terror among the common people, and it was a great cause of pride among the princes and princesses to be allowed to touch it. It was very expensive to obtain the right to touch it.[2]

Artists also decorated moveable partitions and the façades of houses. They carved poles (wrongly called "totem poles") and made ritual instruments. Above all, it was their responsibility to design, fashion, and manipulate the theatrical machines that in this region of North America gave religious ceremonies the appearance of spectacular performances. They took place outdoors or in the vast residences made of wooden boards. These buildings consisted of a single room in which several families lived, and it could accommodate a large number of guests.

An indigenous narrative dating to the nineteenth century describes a session at which the hearth in the center of the room was suddenly flooded, as at the end of *Twilight of the Gods*, with water rising up from the depths. A life-size cetacean surfaced and shook itself, spouting water through its blowholes. Then it dived, the water disappeared, and on the reconstituted floor the hearth fire could be relit.[3]

The inventors and producers of these phenomenal machines were given no margin for error. In 1895 Franz Boas published the account of a ceremony whose star attraction, as it were, was supposed to be the return of a man, who had supposedly been living at the bottom of the sea, to his family. The spectators who gathered on the shore saw a rock rising up and splitting in two, and then the man emerged. The stagehands hidden in the woods maneuvered the contraption from a distance by means of ropes. Twice the operation succeeded. The third time, the ropes became tangled, the artificial rock sank, and the hero drowned. Unfazed, his family announced that he had chosen to live at the bottom of the ocean, and the celebration continued as planned. But after the guests had left, the deceased's parents and those responsible for the disaster bound themselves together and threw themselves into the sea from the top of a cliff.[4]

The story is also told that, to represent onstage a female initiate's return to earth, artists constructed a whale out of seal skins, operating it with ropes to make it swim and dive. In the interest of realism, they came up with the idea of boiling water inside the whale using red-hot stones, so that steam would spout from the blowholes. A stone fell off to one side, burning the skin, and the whale sank. The organizers of the ceremony and the inventors of the machine committed suicide, knowing that otherwise they would be put to death by the keepers of the secret of these rites.[5]

All these narratives come from the Tsimshian Indians, who live on the coast of British Columbia. Their Haida neighbors on the adjacent Queen Charlotte Islands speak of wondrous villages at the bottom of the sea or in the heart of the forests, populated entirely with artists, from whom the Indians who met them learned to paint and carve.[6] These myths too affirm that the fine arts are supernatural in origin. Nevertheless, in these few examples of religious ceremonies, everything from beginning to end is obviously artifice. First there is the solemn session when the initiator claims (but does he not believe it to a certain extent?) to be visited by his supernatural protector: wresting the spirit from his own body, he casts it violently into that of the novice, hidden under a mat, while at the same time a whistle blows, the sonorous emblem of the spirit in question. Then comes the fabrication of the articulated masks and automatons, which are supposed to manifest the presence and actions of the spirits; and finally, the spectacles, like those that were described by some of the last witnesses.

The aesthetic feeling experienced when observing a successful spectacle validated retrospectively the belief in its supernatural origin. Admittedly, it did so even in the minds of the creators and actors for whom that connection had, at best, only a hypothetical reality since they were aware of the tricks: "It was therefore true, since, despite the many difficulties that we ourselves faced, it succeeded all the same." Conversely, a failed spectacle, which brought the deception to light, ran the risk of destroying the conviction that there was a continuity between the human and supernatural worlds. That conviction was all the more necessary in that, in these hierarchical societies, the power of the nobles, the subordination of the common people, and the submission of slaves were sanctioned by the supernatural order on which the social order therefore depended.

We do not inflict physical death (economic and social death perhaps?) on those we consider no-talent artists incapable of elevating us above ourselves. But do we not still establish a link between art and the supernatural? That is the etymological sense of the word "enthusiasm," which we readily use to characterize the emotion we feel in the presence of great works of art. One used to speak of the "divine" Raphael, and, in English, the language of aesthetics includes the expression "out of this world." In that case as well, we need only convert from the literal to the figurative those beliefs or practices that surprise or upset us, to recognize a certain family resemblance to our own.

As it happens, that same region of North America where the artist's condition appears in a rather sinister light—though he is placed high on the social ladder, he is devoted to trickery and is killed or forced to commit suicide if he fails—has provided us with a charming and poetic portrait of the artist. The Tlingit of Alaska, immediate neighbors of the Tsimshian, recount in one of their myths that a young chief of the Queen Charlotte Islands had a wife whom he dearly loved. She fell ill and, despite the care showered on her, she died. Her husband, inconsolable, searched high and low for a sculptor who could reproduce the features of the deceased. No one was able to do so. But a very illustrious sculptor lived in the same village. One day he ran into the widower and told him: "You go from village to village, and you don't find anyone to create a likeness of your wife, am I right? I saw her often when you were walking together. I never studied her face with the idea that one day you'd want a representation of her, but if you'll allow me, I'll do my best."

The sculptor obtained a red-cedar log and set to work. When his carving was completed, he dressed it in the dead woman's clothes and summoned the husband. Filled with joy, he took the statue and asked the sculptor what he owed: "Whatever you like," replied the other, "but I did it out of sympathy for your sorrow, so do not give me too much." The young chief nevertheless paid the sculptor very well, in both slaves and a variety of riches.

An artist so famous that even a prominent man did not dare ask for his favors; who, before setting to work, believed it was normal to have studied his model's physiognomy; who did not allow people to watch him work; whose works were very valuable; and who, on occasion, knew how to act in a humane and disinterested manner: Is that not the ideal portrait of a great painter or sculptor even now? We would certainly like all our artists to be like him. But let us continue with the myth.

The young chief treated the statue as if it were alive. One day, he even had the impression it was moving. All his visitors went into raptures over the resemblance. Much later, he examined the body and observed it had become just like a human one. (The rest can be surmised.) In fact, a little later, the statue emitted a noise like wood cracking. The statue was lifted up and a little red cedar was discovered growing underneath. It was allowed to mature, and that is why the red cedars of Queen Charlotte Islands are so beautiful. When someone goes looking for a beautiful tree and finds one, they say: "It's like the baby of the chief's wife." As for the statue, it barely moved and no one ever heard it speak, but the husband knew through his dreams that it was communicating with him and what it said.[7]

The Tsimshian (from whom the Tlingit, who admired their artistic talents, readily commissioned works) tell the story of the wooden statue differently. It is the widower himself who carves a statue of the deceased. He treats it as if it were alive, pretends to converse with it by asking it questions and providing the answers. Two sisters slip into his hut one day and hide; they see the man kissing and hugging the wooden statue. This makes them laugh: the man discovers them and invites them to dinner. The younger sister eats in moderation, while the elder consumes greedily. Later, while she is sleeping, she is overcome with diarrhea and soils herself. The younger sister and the widower decide to marry, each making a pledge to the other: he will burn the statue and never mention the elder sister's shame; and she will not tell anyone what he was doing with the wooden statue.[8]

The parallelism between the (quantitative) abuse of food and the (qualitative) abuse of sex is striking, since in both cases it is an abuse of communication: to eat in excess and to copulate with a statue as if it were a human being are behaviors that, though in different registers, are comparable. That is especially true in that the languages of the world (including our own, though only metaphorically) often employ the same word for "eat" and "copulate." But the Tlingit myth and the Tsimshian myth do not treat the motif in the same way. The Tsimshian myth finds the confusion between a human being and a wooden statue reprehensible. It is true that the statue is the work of an amateur, not a professional, and we have seen the mystery that surrounded the works of Tsimshian sculptors and painters. To pass off art as life was both their privilege and their obligation. But since the aim of the illusion created by the work of art was to bear witness to the connection between the social order and the supernatural order, it would not have been acceptable for a private individual to make use of that illusion for his personal benefit. In public opinion, represented by the two sisters, the widower's behavior appeared scandalous or at the very least ridiculous.

The Tlingit myth proposes a different conception of the work of art. The widower's behavior does not shock public opinion: everyone rushes to his house to admire the masterpiece. But in this case, the statue is that of a great artist, and (in spite or because of that) it remains halfway between life and art. Plants produce only plants, and a wooden woman can only give birth to a tree. The Tlingit myth makes art an autonomous realm: the work finds its place beyond and on the near side of the artist's intention; the artist loses control of it as soon as he has created it. It will develop in keeping with its own nature. In other words, the way the work of art perpetuates itself is to give birth to other works of art, which to contemporaries appear more alive than those that preceded.

Seen from a millennial vantage point, human passions become indistinguishable from one another. Time adds nothing to and takes nothing away from the love and hatred human beings feel: their commitments, their struggles, their desires. Then and now, they are always the same. If we were to omit at random ten or twenty centuries of history, our knowledge of human nature would not be appreciably affected. The only irreplaceable loss would be that of the works of art those centuries brought into existence. Human beings differ from one another, even exist, only through their works. Like the wooden statue that gave birth to a tree, these works alone provide evidence that, over the course of time, something has really happened among human beings.

7

MONTAIGNE AND AMERICA

It is significant that the quadricentennial of Montaigne's death coincides with the quincentennial of the discovery of America: both are being celebrated this year. Indeed, no one better than Montaigne was able to understand and anticipate the upheavals that the discovery of the New World would bring to the Old World's philosophical, political, and religious ideas.

Previously the general public and even scholars had seemed largely untroubled by the news, however dramatic, that their kind represented only half the human race. The discovery of "an infinite extent of terra firma," as Montaigne said, "not an island or single country, but a division of the world, nearly equal in greatness to that we knew before," did not come as a revelation. It simply confirmed what was known through the Bible and the Greek and Latin authors: there were faraway lands— Eden, Atlantis, the Garden of the Hesperides, the Fortunate Islands— and strange races, which had already been described by Pliny. The customs of the indigenous peoples of the New World offered nothing very new, when compared to those of the exotic nations known to the ancients. Rather, the reports of these customs simply corroborated the ancient accounts. At the dawn of the sixteenth century European consciousness, all the more certain of its knowledge, could withdraw into itself. For Europe, the discovery of America did not inaugurate modern times: it closed a chapter that had begun in the Renaissance with the discovery, judged much more important, of the ancient world through the Greek and Latin works.

Montaigne was born in 1533 and began thinking soon after. His ever-keen curiosity impelled him to learn about the New World. He had two sources: the first Spanish chronicles of the Conquest and the recently published accounts of French travelers who had shared the Indians' life on the coast of Brazil. He was even acquainted with one of these witnesses and, as we know, encountered a few "savages" brought to Rouen by a sailor.

In comparing these sources, Montaigne became aware of a distinction, which Americanists still make, between the great civilizations of Mexico and Peru and the humble cultures of the tropical lowlands: on the one hand, very dense populations that were in every way our equal in their political organization, the magnificence of their cities, and the refinement of their arts; on the other, little village groups with rudimentary industries, which astonished Montaigne for a different reason. He marveled that life in society needed "so little artifice and human patchwork" to exist and maintain itself.

That contrast orients Montaigne's thinking in two ways. For him, the savages of Brazil, or, as he calls them, "my cannibals," raise the issue of the minimal conditions required for life in society to be possible. In other words: What is the nature of the social bond? Preliminary responses are scattered throughout the *Essais*, but it is clear above all that Montaigne, in formulating the problem, laid the foundations on which Hobbes, Locke, and Rousseau would build the entire political philosophy of the seventeenth and eighteenth centuries. The continuity between Montaigne and Rousseau stands out all the more clearly in that the last response to the question, given by Rousseau in the *Social Contract*, proceeds, like Montaigne's initial inquiry, from a reflection on the ethnographic facts (Rousseau elaborated that reflection in his *Discourse on the Origin of Inequality*). It could almost be said that the lessons Montaigne asked of the Indians of Brazil led via Rousseau to the political doctrines of the French Revolution.

The Aztecs and the Incas raised a different problem since their high level of civilization put distance between them and natural laws. They might have been on an equal footing with the Greeks and the Romans: comparable weapons would have made them safe from the "mechanical victories" that breastplates, knives and swords, and firearms allowed the Spanish to enjoy over peoples still backward in that respect. Montaigne thus discovered that a civilization can display internal discordances and that external discordances exist between civilizations.

The New World provides surprising examples of similarities between its practices and our own, past and present. And because we knew nothing of each other, the indigenous peoples of the Americas could not have borrowed them from us, or vice versa. Since other practices differ from one shore of the Atlantic to the other and even contradict each other, no natural foundation for any of them is to be had.

To extricate himself from that difficulty, Montaigne came up with two possible solutions. The first would be to defer to the court of reason, which views all societies—past and present, near or far away—as barbaric, since their disagreements and accidental agreements have no foundation other than custom. The second solution would acknowledge that "every one gives the title of barbarian to everything that is not in use in his own country." Yet there is no belief or custom, however bizarre, shocking, or even revolting it might appear, for which, when it is placed in its context, a well-reasoned argument could not find an explanation. In the first hypothesis, no practice is justified; all practices are justified in the second.

Montaigne thus opens two perspectives on philosophical thought; and even today, philosophers do not seem to have made a firm choice between them. On the one hand, the philosophy of the Enlightenment subjects all historical societies to its criticism and cherishes the utopian dream of a rational society. On the other, relativism rejects any absolute criterion by which a culture could allow itself to judge different cultures.

Since Montaigne, and following his example, we have never stopped looking for a way out of that contradiction. In 1992, as we commemorate both the death of the author of the *Essais* and the discovery of the New World, it is important to recall that that discovery did not simply procure us material goods (food, industrial products, medicines) that transformed our civilization from top to bottom. It was also the source—in this case, thanks to Montaigne—of ideas that still provide food for thought, of philosophical problems that he was the first to raise. They have lost none of their urgency for contemporary thought—on the contrary. But over the last four centuries, no one has managed to analyze them more lucidly and in more depth than Montaigne in his *Essais*.

8

MYTHIC THOUGHT AND

SCIENTIFIC THOUGHT

Scientific knowledge has advanced more over the course of the twentieth century than it had in two thousand years. It is a curious paradox, however, that the more progress science has made, the more modest the philosophical reflections on science have proved to be. In the seventeenth century, philosophers such as Locke and Descartes had become convinced that the knowledge that comes to us through the senses is deceptive. Behind what we perceive as colors, sounds, and odors, nothing exists but extension and motion. Or at least, the substance of reality was believed to lie therein. A century later, Kant would denounce that illusion, claiming that space and time are also forms that our sensibility takes. The human mind imposes constraints on the world, and if the mind aspires to reason beyond its own limits, it runs up against insoluble contradictions. But that stricture also constitutes our strength: by definition, the world as we perceive it obeys the rules of our logic, since that perception is merely the refraction of an unknowable reality through the mind's architecture.

Since the birth of astrophysics and quantum physics, we must renounce even that claim because science in its new guise confronts us with an incompatibility between what we believe it is possible to know and the rules regulating how our thought process functions. The idea that the universe has a history and that it began with what is conventionally called the Big Bang restores the reality of time and space, but at the same time it obliges us to admit—if this expression were not monstrously contradictory—that there was a time when time did not yet exist, an embryonic universe that was not already in space, since space is said to have appeared along with it. And when astrophysicists explain to the layman (that is, to all of us) that the universe has a known diameter of about ten billion light years, that our galaxy and its neighbors are moving within it at a speed of six hundred kilometers a second, and so on, we must confess that for ordinary people these are empty words and that we are unable to visualize what they represent.

We are told that, on the scale of the infinitely small, a particle and even an atom can be both here and somewhere else, everywhere and nowhere, that it can behave sometimes like a wave and sometimes like a corpuscle. All these propositions have a meaning for the scientist because they stem from mathematical calculations and experiments so complicated that he alone can interpret them. They remain untranslatable into ordinary language, however, because they violate the laws of logical argument, and in the first place the principle of identity.

There is no denying it: like the most extravagant mythic constructions, phenomena that belong to orders of magnitude—large or small—whose existence was long unimagined run counter to common sense. For the nonspecialist, and even more so for the man in the street, the world that physicists attempt to describe for their own purposes reconstitutes an equivalent of sorts to what our remote ancestors conceived as a supernatural world, where everything happens differently than in the ordinary world, usually backward. The ancients and (closer to our own time) peoples without writing invented myths in an attempt to imagine that supernatural world. Ironically, in so doing they sometimes prefigured fables that physicists now invent when they try to make the results of their research and the hypotheses they derive from it accessible to the rest of us.

Here is a lovely example, which involves an amusing transposition to the macroscopic level of phenomena that quantum physics describes at the microscopic level. A myth of the Seneca Indians (one of the five nations composing the Iroquois confederacy) includes a curious episode. A girl agrees to marry a man who, she knows, is the son of a powerful witch, and she follows him to his mother's village: "The husband walked in the lead, and they arrived at a point where the path divided into two trails forming a sort of oblong ring that closed farther along. To her great surprise, the woman saw her husband split in two, and each of the two bodies followed one of the trails. She was astounded by that, not knowing which path she herself ought to take. Fortunately [the myth does not say what would have happened otherwise], she chose the one on the right and soon observed that the two trails joined and that her husband's two bodies once again merged at that point. Hence the origin of that strange individual's name, so they say: it means 'they are two paths running parallel.'" A grammatical plural therefore designates a single being.

The Iroquois, then, conceived a world—different, to be sure, from that of ordinary experience—where a body behaves sometimes like a refracting wave, sometimes like a particle that retains its individuality. This episode is part of a myth too long and complicated to describe in detail here. Suffice it to say that the protagonists, some of them twins, spend their time losing, finding again, borrowing, or exchanging one or both of their eyes, as if vision, which can be monocular or binocular, were a model provided by nature for an operation that remains identical to itself whether it passes through a single channel or through two at once.

This story of a man who splits in two when two paths are offered him bears an astonishing resemblance to the fables that physicists concoct when, in books for the general public, they want to help us understand how a cluster of particles passing through either one or two slits in a screen behaves sometimes like a wave train and sometimes like corpuscles.

In making that comparison, I refrain from engaging in mysticism. Nothing allows us to create or perpetuate confusion between archaic forms of thought and scientific thought. In the realm of experience, one is valid, the others are not, even though they draw from the same lexicon to express themselves in ordinary language. The idea that matter is made up of atoms dates back to remote antiquity, but in that case it was a gratuitous hypothesis that remained unverifiable by the only means of observation available, the sense organs. It would acquire validity only when applied to phenomena and events so small that for a long time they remained inaccessible. That is even more true for the duality between the wave and the corpuscle.

In both cases, however, what is interesting is that pure intellectual speculation could offer a representation—preliminary, crude, and confused, to be sure—of an order of reality that human beings were in no position to know.

Greek philosophy from the earliest days, as it was outlined twenty-five hundred years ago by the pre-Socratics, prompts the same order of reflections. One thinker claimed that water constitutes the primordial reality from which everything emerged; another says it was fire, and a third, air. Some claimed that reality originally formed a homogeneous whole, others that it was and continues to be composed of atoms. These same philosophers inquired into the nature of existence and alteration, immobility and change, and so on. In so doing, they explored concepts without any reference to reality and were concerned only with seeing how far they could pursue their intellectual gymnastics. They engaged in a systematic inventory of the *possibilities* delimited by the mind's constraints. Their philosophical reflections did not deal with the world but rather set about mapping mental frameworks. They drew up a table, some of whose boxes would be filled in through the future progress of knowledge, while others would remain vacant, temporarily or permanently. The control experiment, testing of the facts, was absent. The mind, not yet disciplined by research, became intoxicated by its own power and by the discovery of its virtualities.

An exemplary anecdote on this subject is recounted by Plutarch in his *Table Talks*. Its hero is one of the most famous pre-Socratic philosophers. One day when Democritus was eating a fig, he found it had the flavor of honey, and he asked his servant where the fruit had come from. She indicated an orchard, and Democritus wanted her to take him there immediately so that he could consider and examine the place and there discover the cause of that sweetness. "Don't bother," said the servant, "because, without paying attention, I put those figs in a vase that had contained honey." "Your telling me that makes me angry," Democritus replied. "I intend to pursue my idea, and I will seek the cause as if the sweetness came from the fig itself."

According to tradition, Democritus widely practiced empirical observation. In the present case, his first impulse led him in that direction, but he could not resist the pleasure he had promised himself to exercise his mind, even in a vacuum or on the basis of false premises. That, Plutarch observes, is a secondary detail, once one is presented with "a subject and a subject matter worth discoursing on."

Ever since humanity has existed, always and everywhere "pursuing one's idea" has been a constant occupation. That exercise brings human beings satisfaction; they find an intrinsic interest in it, not even asking where that exploration will lead. It is true—as demonstrated by the history of scientific thought and, especially, of mathematics—that the exploration of the powers of the mind always leads somewhere, even if several centuries or millennia go by before the fantastic-sounding ideas are revealed to be simply a reflection of a long-hidden level of the real world.

The myths that human beings fed on for so long may amount to the same thing: a systematic and never useless exploration of the resources of the imagination. Myths depict all sorts of creatures and events, absurd or contradictory when compared to ordinary experience, which will cease to be totally meaningless only at a level incommensurate with the level where the myths were first elaborated. It is because these myths are already inscribed—as a dotted line so to speak—in the mind's architecture, which is "of the world," that one day or another the images of the world set forth by myths will prove to be adequate to that world and well-suited to illustrate aspects of it.

It is therefore easier to understand why Niels Bohr, one of the fathers of quantum physics, invited his contemporaries to turn to ethnologists and poets as a means of overcoming the contradictions of their discipline. As he acknowledged forty years ago at a conference where ethnologists were gathered, "the traditional differences between human cultures resemble in many respects the different but equivalent ways that physical experience can be described." Only the images of a wave and a corpuscle, employed simultaneously, allow us to grasp the properties of a single object; in the same way, ethnologists form an idea of culture, a universal human idea, only through beliefs, customs, and institutions that contradict one another and are often self-contradictory.

As for the poets, they make an original and synthetic use of language to reach truths located at a deeper level than that of ordinary experience: they multiply perspectives to define the outlines of an object that remains elusive, and they juxtapose words with incompatible meanings (the old grammarians called them oxymorons). Myths could be included as well since every myth allows for a plurality of variants. Through different and often contradictory images, these variants seek to make perceptible a structure that escapes direct efforts at description.

Scientific thought in its most modern form therefore invites us to recognize that in language, and probably from the very first, metaphor and analogy have enjoyed a legitimate existence, as Vico affirmed. He denied they were "ingenious inventions of writers."[1] The parallel evolution of the human and natural sciences leads in the same direction. It too encourages us to see figurative language as a fundamental mode of thought, which moves us closer to reality rather than cutting us off from it, as was once believed. Back in the eighteenth century,

Vico denounced "two common errors of the grammarians: that prose speech is proper speech, and poetic speech improper; and that prose speech came first, and afterwards speech in verse." According to him, what was true at the beginning of humankind may now be becoming true once again.

9

WE ARE ALL CANNIBALS

Until 1932 the mountains in the interior of New Guinea remained the last totally unknown region on the planet. Formidable natural defenses prevented access to them. Gold prospectors, followed shortly thereafter by missionaries, penetrated them first, but World War II interrupted these attempts. It was only in 1950 that we began to realize that this vast territory held almost a million people, speaking different languages that all belonged to the same family. These peoples were unaware of the existence of whites, whom they mistook for deities or ghosts. Their customs, their beliefs, and their social organization would open up an unimagined field of study to ethnologists.

And not only to ethnologists. In 1956 an American biologist, Dr. Carleton Gajdusek, discovered an unknown disease in the region. In small populations distributed among some 160 villages over a territory of about 250 square miles, about thirty-five thousand individuals in all, one person in a hundred died every year of a degenerative disease of the central nervous system. It manifested itself as uncontrollable shaking (hence its name, "kuru," which means "tremble" or "shiver" in the language of the principal group concerned) and a gradual loss of coordination of voluntary movements, followed by multiple infections. Gajdusek, having at first believed that the malady was genetic in origin, demonstrated that it was caused by a slow-acting, particularly resistant virus, which no one was ever able to isolate.

This was the first time that a degenerative disease caused by a slow-acting virus had been identified in humans, but animal diseases such as scrapie in sheep and mad cow disease, which recently ravaged Great Britain, are very similar. And in human beings, another degenerative ailment of the nervous system, Creutzfeldt-Jakob disease, has appeared sporadically throughout the world. In showing that, as with kuru, apes could be infected with Creutzfeldt-Jakob, Gajdusek demonstrated that kuru was identical to that disease (a genetic predisposition is not ruled out). For that discovery, he received the Nobel Prize in Medicine for 1976.

In the case of kuru, the genetic hypothesis was not a good match for the statistics. The disease struck women and young children much more often than adult men, so much so that in the villages most affected, there was only one woman for two or three, or sometimes even four, men. Kuru, which seems to have appeared at the beginning of the twentieth century, therefore also had sociological consequences: a reduction in the rate of polygamy, a larger proportion of single men and widowers caring for families, greater freedom for women in the choice of a husband.

But if kuru was infectious in origin, the carrier(s) of the virus and the reason for its uneven distribution between the sexes and among different age groups still had to be found. Nothing turned up as a result of inquiries into diet and the unhealthy living conditions of the huts where the women and children resided (their husbands and fathers lived apart from them in a collective house; sexual relations took place in the forest or in gardens).

When ethnologists entered the region in turn, they advanced a different hypothesis. Before the groups that had fallen victim to kuru had come under the control of the Australian administration, they had indulged in cannibalism. The act of eating the corpse of certain close relatives was a means of demonstrating affection and respect for them. The flesh, viscera, and brains were cooked; the bones were ground up and served with vegetables. The women were in charge of cutting up the corpses and of the other culinary operations, and they were particularly fond of these macabre meals. It may be supposed that they became infected while handling contaminated brains and that they infected their young children through bodily contact.

It seems that these cannibalistic practices began in the region around the same time that kuru made its appearance. Furthermore, ever since the presence of whites put an end to cannibalism, the incidence of kuru has steadily declined, and the disease has now almost vanished. A causal link may therefore exist. Caution is required, however, since the cannibalistic practices, described by indigenous informants with a remarkable wealth of details, had already disappeared when the investigations began. No direct observation or experience in the field allows us to say that the problem is definitively solved.

*
* *

As it happens, in the last few months in France, Great Britain, and Australia, the press has become fascinated with the cases of Creutzfeldt-Jakob disease (identical, as I said, to kuru) that broke out following injections of hormone extracted from human pituitary glands (the pituitary is a small gland located at the base of the brain) or grafts from the brain membranes of humans. The first treatment is used to combat growth disorders in young children; the second, female infertility. Several deaths resulting from infertility treatments were reported in Great Britain, New Zealand, and the United States; other fatalities occurred more recently in France, among children treated with growth hormone extracted from human brains, which were probably improperly sterilized. There is talk of a scandal comparable to the one that, on a larger scale, distressed the French public when blood became contaminated by the AIDS virus. As in that case, lawsuits have been filed.

The hypothesis advanced by ethnologists, and accepted by doctors and biologists—that kuru, a disease confined to a few small exotic populations, had its origin in cannibalism—is therefore dramatically illustrated in the Western world. Here and there, similar diseases may have been communicated to women and children who incorporated, by different pathways of course, human cerebral materials. One case does not prove the other, but there is a striking analogy between them.

Some may protest against that comparison. But what essential difference is there between the oral route and the blood route, between ingestion and injection, for introducing into an organism a little of the substance of another? People will say it is the bestial appetite for human flesh that makes cannibalism horrible. They will then have to restrict their condemnation to a few extreme cases and omit from the definition of cannibalism other attested cases, where it is imposed as a religious obligation, often performed with repugnance—revulsion even—expressed as faintness and vomiting. The distinction some would be tempted to make between a barbaric and superstitious custom on the one hand, a practice grounded in scientific knowledge on the other, would hardly be convincing either. Many uses of substances drawn from the human body, scientific from the standpoint of the ancient pharmacopoeia, are considered by us to be superstitions. And after a few years modern medicine itself proscribes treatments, formerly believed to be effective, because they have turned out to be useless if not harmful. The distinction appears to be less sharp than one would like to imagine.

Nevertheless, prevailing opinion continues to see the practice of cannibalism as a monstrosity, an aberration of human nature so inconceivable that certain authors, victims of that prejudice, have come to deny that cannibalism ever existed. It is the invention of travelers and ethnologists, they say. The proof: over the course of the nineteenth and twentieth centuries, ethnologists produced countless accounts from throughout the world, but nowhere was a scene of cannibalism directly observed. (I leave aside those exceptional cases where people, about to starve to death, were reduced to eating their already-dead companions, since what is being disputed is the existence of cannibalism as a custom or institution.)

In *The Man-Eating Myth* (Oxford University Press, 1979), a brilliant but superficial book that enjoyed great success with an ill-informed readership, W. Arens attacks in particular the received ideas about kuru. If stories of cannibalism are fables that, as he claims (111–12), emerged from a complicity between researchers and their indigenous informants, there is no more reason to believe that cannibalism was the source of kuru in New Guinea than there would be to believe that Creutzfeldt-Jakob disease is transmitted in Europe by the same means: a grotesque hypothesis that no one had ever advanced.

Yet, as we have just seen, it is precisely the indisputable reality of the second case (Creutzfeldt-Jakob) that, though not providing proof, confers increased likelihood on the first.

*

*   *

No serious ethnologist disputes the reality of cannibalism, but they all know as well that it cannot be reduced to its most brutal form, which consists of killing enemies in order to eat them. That custom certainly existed in Brazil—to confine ourselves to a single example—where a few ancient travelers and Portuguese Jesuits, who lived for years among the Indians in the sixteenth century and spoke their language, were very eloquent witnesses to it.

Alongside exocannibalism, a place must be made for endocannibalism, which consists of consuming, in large or very small quantities, whether fresh or in its putrefied or mummified state, the flesh—raw, cooked, or charred—of deceased relatives. On the border of Brazil and Venezuela, the Yanomami Indians, the unfortunate victims of abuse from the gold prospectors who invaded their territory, even now consume the bones, ground up beforehand, of their dead.

Cannibalism can be practiced to meet nutritional needs (in times of scarcity or because of a taste for human flesh); it can be a political act (punishment for criminals or revenge against one's enemies); it can have a magical function (assimilation of the virtues of the deceased or, on the contrary, the casting out of their souls); or it can be part of a ritual (a religious cult, a feast of the dead or coming-of-age ceremony, or a rite to assure agricultural prosperity). Finally, it can be therapeutic, as attested by many prescriptions in ancient medicine and in Europe itself in the not-so-remote past. Injections of pituitary gland and grafts of human brain matter indisputably belong to that last category, as do organ transplants, which have become common practice.

So varied are the modalities of cannibalism, so diverse its real or supposed functions, that we may come to doubt whether the notion of cannibalism as it is currently employed can be defined in a relatively precise manner. It dissolves or dissipates as soon as one attempts to grasp it. Cannibalism in itself has no objective reality. It is an ethnocentric category: it exists only in the eyes of the societies that proscribe it. All flesh, whatever its provenance, is a cannibal food in Buddhism, which believes in the unity of life. Conversely, in Africa and Melanesia, some groups made human flesh one food among others, if not at times the best, the most respectable, the only one, they said, that "has a name."

Authors who deny the present and past existence of cannibalism claim that the notion was invented to widen the gap between "savages" and the civilized. Supposedly, we falsely attribute to them revolting customs and beliefs in order to clear our consciences and confirm our belief in our superiority.

Let us reverse that tendency and seek to perceive the facts of cannibalism in all their ramifications. Employing extraordinarily diverse modalities and ends, depending on the time and place, the practice always entails intentionally introducing into the bodies of human beings parts or substances from other human bodies. The notion of cannibalism, thus exorcised, will now appear rather commonplace. Jean-Jacques Rousseau saw the origin of social life in the sentiment that impels us to identify with others. And after all, the most simple means to identify others with oneself is to eat them.

In the last analysis, if travelers to distant lands have easily—and not without indulgence—bowed to the evidence of cannibalism, it is because in that generalized form, the only one that allows us to embrace the totality of the phenomenon, the concept of cannibalism and its direct or indirect applications belong to all societies. As demonstrated by the parallel I traced between Melanesian customs and our own practices, we can even go so far as to say that it also exists among us.

10

AUGUSTE COMTE AND ITALY

Auguste Comte, the founder of positivism, granted an increasingly large place to Italy as his philosophy of science yielded in importance to the establishment of a new religion. Granted, the religious idea, the only one capable of disciplining progress by means of order, was never absent from his system. In the organization of his church, he had first considered giving preeminence to the Germanic nations (after France, that is), where Protestantism and the free examination of conscience had favored the rise of rational thought. The Great Priest of Humanity would have his seat in Paris, assisted by a college composed of eight Frenchmen, seven Englishmen, six Germans, five Italians, and four Spaniards. The Italians would represent, respectively, Piedmont, Lombardy, Tuscany, the Roman Republic, and the Neapolitan region.

He invokes that plan in the first volume of *Système de politique positive* (*System of Positive Polity*), published in 1851. It had been written in the preceding months: for Comte, the writing process was immediately followed by publication; he meditated for a long time, then wrote in one sitting and never reread what he had written. The book was composed, therefore, on the eve of Cavour's coming to power. After that, however, Comte announced a different plan. In the fourth and last volume, published in 1854, he explains that, though Protestantism had played a role in the birth of Enlightenment philosophy, it had kept that philosophy from advancing past the stage of metaphysical thought. In the political order, moreover, Protestantism, unable by its very essence to give rise to a spiritual power, placed religion under the control of temporal power: for example, in England with the Anglican Church and in Germany with the Protestant states.

In Comte's eyes, by contrast, the separation of the two powers, the spiritual and the temporal, had been the major success of medieval Catholicism, and the first task of the Religion of Humanity would be to reinstate it. In that respect, the nations of Western Europe that had been shielded from Protestantism and that best preserved "the felicitous moral culture of the Middle Ages" would also be best able to reconstitute the ideal of temporally independent nations "linked spiritually, however, through a freely-agreed-upon aggregation."

In the historical evolution of the West, the stage of Protestant negativism, at which Germany and England were arrested, and that of Voltairean deism, which had replaced it in France, were not at all inevitable. Italy and even Spain could easily skip them, just as France had skipped Calvinism. To make up for their apparent delay, southern Europeans would proceed directly from Catholicism to positivism. The Religion of Humanity, liberated from the theological frame of mind and the belief in revelation, would be a new "Catholicism," in the etymological sense of an aspiration to universality.

As a result, the order of precedence among nations changed. France remained the central nation, but Italy was second, followed by Spain and Great Britain, with Germany in last place. With the Pontiff of Humanity at the center, each country would be represented by a national Superior; three others (not initially foreseen) would represent "the West's colonial expansions."

Essentially, Italy was to have priority over Spain because its military inferiority, resulting from its lack of concentrated political power, kept it pure of all colonization: "often oppressed, the Italian people were never the oppressor." Conversely, the Iberian nations had retained from their colonialist past oppressive tendencies that, Comte feared, would disturb the harmony of the Western world.

The lack of concentrated political power was all to the advantage of the Italians. Comte said he was convinced that aspirations for national unity, so strong in that nineteenth-century environment, were confined to the literati—to intellectuals, we would now say—and did not have roots in the common people. Positivism would liberate Italy from the Austrian yoke but, once that goal was achieved, the country would not heed "those spiritual guides of the population who have never ceased to yearn for its ancient domination and even to dream of its universal return." More than a century in advance, then, Comte foresaw what the future consequences of an intensification of national feeling could be in Italy and Spain. He had seen it in France during his lifetime, the Napoleonic dictatorship having arisen from the nationalist fervor of the Revolution.

In Italy, national unity would be a reactionary yearning, even worse than the artificial aggregations visible in the country at the time (1850, let us not forget), "especially the one whose multiple names indicate sufficiently its heterogeneity, primarily in the jumbled group that assembles five incompatible states in the north."

*
* *

Comte is in fact deeply hostile to the states. He sees them as the products of a martial Old Regime that, prior to the advent of positive science, "could not undertake the conquest of a world that seemed as invincible as it was inexplicable, and where every partial association strove above all to subjugate the others."

The new religion would of course need intermediate bodies, which could be called homelands, to intervene between these families and humanity. Comte conceives of them as free and lasting associations much smaller than states, founded on respect for local diversities, each one a spontaneous gathering of the rural populations around a dominant city. That was the situation prevailing in the Middle Ages, the one that Italy, better than other places, had been able to preserve.

France would set an example for the other countries. It would initiate its own dismemberment, breaking up into seventeen small republics. Western Europe would have seventy and the world as a whole five hundred, each composed on average of three hundred thousand families, on the same order of magnitude, therefore, as Tuscany, Sicily, and Sardinia. Was Comte prophetic? We now see here and there, in Europe and the rest of the world, minorities rising up to demand their rights, an aggravation of particularism that, in certain cases at least, has already led to the dismemberment of states.

It was precisely because, in about 1850, Italy still lived under a system of political decomposition that it was closer to the normal state of human societies. Provided it would consent to give precedence to intellectual and moral development over political unrest, Italy, more than the northern nations, would be able to proceed directly from Catholicism to positivism and to fulfill all the conditions proper to medieval society.

These conditions, Comte continues, belonged more to the realm of sentiment than to that of reason, given that they were primarily moral in nature. And it was in the area of sentiment and morality that the genius of Italy asserted its preeminence. Comte praises Italy for having always placed art before science. He all but worships the man he consistently calls "the incomparable Dante," in part, no doubt, for personal reasons: in his eyes, the Platonic love he felt for Clotilde de Vaux, whom he made the Madonna of positivist religion after her premature death, reproduced across the span of centuries Dante's love for Beatrice, Petrarch's love for Laura: "It is through women that positivism must penetrate into Italy and Spain."

For the last seven years, he wrote in 1853 (hence since 1846, the year of Clotilde's death), he had read a canto of Dante every evening. Since the pontificate of the Religion of Humanity would have its seat in France, the other states would have to give up national possession of noble remains: Dante's coffin, already stolen from Florence by

Ravenna, would be "better honored in the principal seat of the universal religion" and would thus be transferred to Paris.

For the positive religion to extend to the entire planet, a common language would have to be bestowed on it, a language necessarily developed by the common people—not an artificial language but an already-existing language that would meet with unanimous approval. What language could fulfill that requirement if not Italian, the most cultured language of poetry and music, the one fashioned by the most peaceful and the most aesthetic population, the only one pure of all colonization?

Positivism would thus merge the five Western languages—French, English, German, Spanish, and Italian—"under the presidency of the most musical one." The language of Dante and Ariosto, first rendered sacred for the needs of the Religion of Humanity, would be the universal language. In short, if Comte had achieved his ends, at international assemblies you would hear nothing but Italian rather than American English.

With its language, Italy would make its contribution to the new world order. Then, too, that language alone would be able to provide an aesthetic complement to the concrete Religion of Humanity. It would fall to an Italian of genius who had converted to positivism to compose an epic, a great poem that would celebrate the outcome of the Western revolution "just as Dante's incomparable composition instituted its beginning."

This poem, titled *Humanity*, which Comte confesses he is incapable of writing, would nevertheless be inspired by the "cerebral crisis" he suffered in his youth. The result would represent decisive progress vis-à-vis Dante's work, which, as a mere excursion from one world to another, appears static: it renders a *vision*. Comte, by contrast, would provide the material for a *lived experience*. During his period of madness, he followed a course opposite to that which humanity had traveled over the course of history: he regressed from the positive stage to the metaphysical stage, then to the polytheistic stage, and finally to the fetishistic stage. After that descent, which lasted three months, he gradually climbed back up over five months' time. That dynamic opposition would dictate the poem's structure. The poem would consist of thirteen cantos: a preliminary one would idealize cerebral unity; the next three would be devoted to mental decline, from the relative to the absolute, "always yearning for complete harmony without ever being able to achieve it." The following eight cantos would show the heart and mind gradually rising toward positive unity, and the thirteenth would idealize an existence that had returned to normal.

Through that work, the Italian genius would fulfill its mission, both psychological and social. The positive religion highlights the character of that genius, more poetic than philosophical, a synthesis that "the most aesthetic of all populations" would be called upon to realize.

*   *   *

The preeminent place given to Italy, to its arts and language, sheds light on one of the most significant aspects of Comte's thought. He conceived progress as three phases leading humanity successively from the theological state to the metaphysical state, and finally, to the positive state. In his thinking, however, no phase abolishes the one that precedes it. Even while making a decisive leap forward, each phase, and especially the last one, rehabilitates and takes control of what constituted the richness of the previous state(s).

It was because Italy and, to a lesser degree, Spain had preserved archaic traits that they would place in the service of the positive state an emotional richness that could not have been produced on its own. Comte goes even further, proclaiming that, once science has been liberated from all anthropomorphism, the poetic and aesthetic resources of human thought at its beginnings, which would now pose no danger for science, could be reintegrated into collective beliefs and practices.

Humanity, having attained the positive state, would not turn its back on the fetishism of the early ages (the primitive mentality, we would now call it). On the contrary, it would be able once more to make a place for fetishism, as Dante had done: his work establishes not an opposition between the two historical ways of representing heaven (as the seat of astrological influences, a pagan heritage; and as the providence of a supreme God, as in Christianity) but rather a harmony.

Comte is still thinking of Dante in his last work, *Synthèse subjective* (*Subjective Synthesis*), only one volume of which was written and published before his death. In it he articulates the rules that, in this last state of his thought, apply both to philosophical and poetic works and are inspired by a concrete arithmetic attributing a symbolic value to prime numbers: "Since the stanzas or groups now have seven lines, their structure and succession will combine the two modes proper to Italian epic, joining the unity of the octave and the continuity of the tercet, through cross rhymes and linkages between strophes. The first line of a stanza always rhymes with the last line of the previous one [actually the next-to-last line, it appears], whose final consonance is thus tripled like the other two."

Although in 1854 Comte felt incapable of composing on his own the poem *Humanity*, for which he aspired only to supply the material to an Italian of genius, a new Dante, twelve years later he believed it possible to give a poetic form to his philosophical thought and even to merge poetry and philosophy. The first volume of *Synthèse subjective*, which has nearly eight hundred pages, is a gigantic composition that follows the rules of metrics. Every sentence has a maximum of 250 letters. The book is divided into seven chapters, each composed of three parts, themselves divided into seven sections comprising seven groups of sentences. One has only to replace the sentence as basic element with the poetic line to discover cantos divided into stanzas, as practiced by "the most aesthetic population." Here again the reference is to Dante.

As an equivalent to rhyme, Comte invented an incredibly complicated play of assonance. Every paragraph has, as a catchword of sorts, a word borrowed from one of the five Western languages, plus Latin and possibly Greek. The letters of the catchword provide, in order, the initial letters (which themselves have other catchwords) of each sentence. The entire work thus rests on a combination of emblematic words, initial letters, and phonetic correspondences in the manner—Comte himself makes the comparison—of simple, double, triple, quadruple, and even quintuple acrostics, which were in vogue among the Renaissance poets.

But what Comte does not seem to see is that this procedure, when distended over eight hundred pages, tens of thousands of lines, and hundreds of thousands of words, loses all its appeal. The reader no longer perceives any link between content and form. More precisely, since the content of a philosophical work consists of abstract ideas, everything in it is reduced to form. Comte is obscurely aware of this when he reserves the aesthetic enjoyment of his construct for an elite of initiates: "I would therefore be surprised," he writes, "if it were sensed immediately by any but a few all-round positivists, that is, by the religious, to whom it offers a universal and permanent application of their sacred formula, by combining love with order for progress."

In that sense we can say that Comte, often a prophet but in this case in spite of himself, prefigures what has become a common illusion among many contemporary artists. Whether in poetry, painting, or especially music, it consists of believing that, because every work capable of eliciting an aesthetic emotion has a structure, one need only invent and set in motion a structure for an aesthetic emotion to result. We may marvel at Comte's ingenuity, but the work of the intelligence does not create an aesthetic emotion unless it has its starting point in sensibility.

Comte's admiration for Italy and for Dante was not without reservation. Dante's art, like that of the Renaissance painters who followed, suffers from having been born at a time when the feudal order and the ambition for universality—which had made for the greatness of medieval Catholicism—were already drawing to a close: "Art therefore had to idealize beliefs and mores, whose perceived decline kept the poet and the public from attaining the intimate convictions demanded by any great aesthetic impression."

And Comte continues: "Dante's incomparable composition is characterized by the extraordinary coincidence between two contrary impulses. That anti-aesthetic situation, at a time when everything was being transformed and even distorted before it could be idealized, obliged art to open up to an artificial solution by seeking in memories of the ancient type those fixed and pronounced mores it could not find around itself."

In thus judging the spirit of the Italian Renaissance at its beginnings, Comte, as always, proved to be a forceful analyst and a great philosopher of history. But he had no artistic education, which no doubt explains why he felt uncomfortable when confronted with the wealth and overabundance of works produced at that time. In some sense, he saw them as a pathological phenomenon, an effect of vain efforts to overcome contradictions. "The admirable Italian culture," he wrote, "has until now often been regarded as excessive because it failed to find its true destiny."

Even if he had converted Italy to positivism and thus given its art "its true destiny," we may doubt whether he would have known to propose something other than the bizarre apparatus of rules in the form of riddles, *bout-rimés*, and alliterations by which what he imagined to be his poetic faculties were exercised on the eve of his death. Curiously, that illusion made Comte a precursor of the eccentric avant-garde that flourished at the end of the nineteenth century and throughout the twentieth, rather than the worthy successor of Dante, though he believed that one of the missions assigned to his own genius was to receive and perpetuate Dante's legacy. But did not Italy *also* produce Futurism?

11

VARIATIONS ON THE THEME OF

A PAINTING BY POUSSIN

"A philosopher painter," Poussin's contemporaries called him. The monumental exhibition taking place in Paris until January 2 [1995] to celebrate the four hundredth anniversary of his birth convinces us that even today his paintings offer food for thought.

Consider the example of *Echo and Narcissus*, also called *The Death of Narcissus*, an illustration of an ancient myth whose poetic and symbolic charge is still alive for us. Have not the terms "narcissistic" and "narcissism" become part of ordinary language?

It is in the first place the painting's composition that holds our attention. All the lines diverge. Narcissus's legs are spread on the right, and his arms are askew. The bodies of the other two figures, the nymph Echo and the putto bearing a funeral torch, are leaning in opposite directions. That deviation from the vertical is replicated by the branches of the tree that occupies the upper half of the painting. By visual means, these divergent orientations evoke the acoustical phenomenon of the echo, which gradually removes itself from the call or cry that produced it, until it is lost in the distance. As in one of Baudelaire's best-known sonnets, that suggestive correspondence between different sense impressions marks the painting with a melancholy, a nostalgic sadness accentuated by the uniformity of the colors.

Under the entry "Écho," the Littré dictionary assembles quotations from good authors. Numbering about a dozen, they are all imbued with yearning and sweetness. The principal virtue they acknowledge in the echo, it seems, is that, by means of repetition, it revives the precious memory of words or songs that are no longer. In his own dictionary, Furetière—who, like Poussin, lived in the seventeenth century—confines himself to a single example, which is no less instructive: "Unhappy lovers will make their complaints to the echo." The technical uses of the word preserve that tone. In music, "echo" is defined as a softer repetition: "Echoes on the organ are very agreeable," says Furetière. In poetry, the echo is used to produce a recherché effect.

The positive value that Western thought grants to the echo—countless examples could be found outside France as well—is not universal, however. I offer as proof the negative value that the Indians of North and South America assign to the echo in their myths. Echo appears in the form of an evil demon who pushes those who question him to the limit by obstinately repeating their questions. When the speaker becomes angry, Echo brutally beats him, leaving him an invalid; or he binds the speaker with human intestines, which he possesses by the basketful. Other traditions attribute to Old Lady Echo the power to cause cramps, which is also a way of paralyzing her victims.

It is true that Echo sometimes proves helpful. An ogre questions him about the direction taken by an escaped fugitive. Echo delays him by repeating his questions instead of providing him with information. Whatever the adversary, then, Echo immobilizes him or slows him down. Far from being, as in Europe, in complicity with the person speaking, far from agreeing with the feelings that drive him, the American Echo always has the function of erecting an obstacle or of obstructing.

It is clear where the opposition lies. For us, the echo awakens yearnings. For Amerindians, it is the cause of misunderstanding: a response is expected, and the echo is not one. And the two terms are at odds with each other. Yearning is an excess of communication with oneself: one suffers from remembering things that would be better forgotten. Conversely, misunderstanding can be defined as a failure of communication, this time with others.

That argument appears abstract and theoretical, the kind for which Baudelaire feared he would be reproached one day "because it may make the mistake of bringing mathematical methods to mind." Nevertheless, it faithfully reflects what the myths on the origin of the echo say in the Old and New Worlds.

The Greeks and the Inuit both personify the echo as a young girl who has been turned into stones. According to one version of the Greek myth, she rejected the god Pan because she was still yearning for Narcissus, with whom she was in love and who, hostile to love, pushed her away. In the Inuit myth, it is she who was hostile to love and marriage; her people therefore abandoned her. Repentant, and having sought refuge atop a cliff, she issued marriage proposals to the men she saw from a distance fishing in their kayaks, but they did not believe her or did not understand her. Yearning, the driving force of the Greek myth, is here reversed into misunderstanding. And the reversal continues to the end: whereas the Greek nymph is dismembered by shepherds whom Pan has driven mad in an act of revenge, the Inuit heroine dismembers herself and turns the pieces of her body into rocks. That is the same as the Greek heroine's fate—intentionally produced in one case; passively suffered in the other.

*
*   *

Things are not so simple, however (they rarely are when one is comparing myths). Although the myth of Narcissus places the emphasis on the theme of yearning, the theme of misunderstanding is not absent. Consider how Ovid recounts the story of Echo and Narcissus in book 3 of *The Metamorphoses*. Desperately in love, Echo follows him deep into the woods. But she is unable to take the initiative because Juno, to punish her for having sought to distract her with her chatter while

Jupiter was pursuing his amorous adventures, had condemned Echo to being unable to speak first or to being silent when someone talked to her, and to repeating only the last words of the voice she heard.

When Narcissus, separated from his companions, becomes worried and calls out: "Is there anyone near me?" Echo repeats: " . . . me." "Come!" says Narcissus, and she calls to him in turn. When no one appears, Narcissus is astonished: "Why do you flee me?" he says, and Echo returns his words. "Misled by that voice, which reproduces his own, he replies 'Let us join together.' Echo, in transports of joy, replies, ' . . . Let us join together,' and hurls herself at Narcissus. Upon seeing her, he draws back and exclaims: 'Let me die if I abandon myself to your desires,' and Echo repeats: ' . . . I abandon myself to your desires.'" And so on.

This is a complete misunderstanding, but the opposite of the one for which the American myths make Echo responsible. Here the protagonists, far from accusing each other of incomprehension, imagine they are conversing: Echo believes that Narcissus's words are addressed to her, and he believes that someone is replying to him. For both of them, the misunderstanding does not seem to be one. They attribute to it a positive content. By contrast, that content is always negative in the American myths.

That is not all: the theme of misunderstanding, this time with the same negative content as in the Americas, also exists in the Greek myth, but it has been transferred from the acoustical register to the visual. Narcissus mistakes his reflection in the water for another whose beauty dazzles him and with whom he falls in love (previously, he had rejected both girls and boys). Only after the fact does he discover that the reflection is himself. Desperate upon learning that his love is impossible, he too dies from the consequences of a misunderstanding.

The best proof that we are arriving at a foundation common to the Greek and American myths is that, according to the former, a flower sprouts from the body of Narcissus (it grows near his head in Poussin's painting). Named after him, this flower is the narcissus, *narkissos* in Greek, from *narke*, which means numbness. That was in fact the power attributed to this flower, cherished by the gods of the underworld. The Furies were offered narcissus wreaths and garlands because it was believed they made their victims numb. In that way, the visual misunderstanding to which Narcissus succumbed coincides with the auditory misunderstanding imputable, in the American myths, to the demon Echo, who paralyzes victims by afflicting them with cramps or tying them up with intestines.

It is therefore not surprising that incest, which is a paralysis of matrimonial exchanges, appears in these myths. As with the echo, at issue in incest is always the strange presence of the same where one expected to find the different. One version of the myth of Narcissus recounts that he was in love with his twin sister. She died, and the grief-stricken Narcissus sought to see her image again by contemplating his own reflection in the water. And American myths attribute incestuous desires to a figure who bore a resemblance to the echo in that, instead of replying, he repeated the question. These behaviors were disapproved of, and, the myth concludes, it is since that time that incest has been prohibited.

If the Greek myth expresses through the visual code what the American myths express through the acoustic code, is the reverse also true? Do we find in the Americas visual images of the echo corresponding to the representation the Greeks produced at the auditory level? Only the Indians who live on the Pacific Coast of Canada seem to have produced a plastic representation of the echo. For them, it was a supernatural spirit, whom they depicted on human-looking masks equipped with interchangeable mouths: of the bear, the wolf, the crow, the frog, the fish, the sea anemone, the rock, and so on. The dancer carried these accessories in a basket hanging from his belt and discreetly substituted one for another as the myth unfolded.

Here the echo is no longer characterized by sterile and monotonous repetition, the cause of numbness and paralysis. On the contrary, what these masks of a hundred mouths evoke is the inexhaustible plasticity of the echo, its ever-renewed power to reproduce the most unexpected sounds. The different versions of the Greek myth also contrast these two aspects. Sometimes Echo is guilty and will be able to reproduce only the last part of the words she has heard; sometimes she is innocent and will receive the power to imitate all sounds, a faculty for which the American masks offer a visual illustration.

It is significant that, in one case, the myth places the emphasis on articulated language and, in the other, on music. Indeed, for the Greeks, music, much superior to the spoken word, was a means of communicating with the gods. Echo was too talkative, she misused language, and she would find herself condemned to make minimal use of it. By contrast, it is because Pan not only desired the nymph but was jealous of her musical gifts that he had her torn to pieces and turned her members into rocks, where, thanks to the echo, her song will continue to resonate.

A detour through the Americas has allowed us to identify the common foundation of the myths. The divergences that apparently predominate in Poussin's composition are thereby revealed in all their aspects. Such divergences are inherent in the physical phenomenon of the echo, which seems, paradoxically, both idiotic and capable of the most surprising achievements. Hence the curiosity to which it gives rise, the fascination it has for hikers and tourists. Poussin's painting also makes these divergences manifest in the way the nymph Echo and the little emissary from a supernatural world lean in different directions: one inclined toward the rocky earth, from which she is already nearly indistinguishable, thanks to a uniform grisaille; the other inclined toward the sky, where the only gleam of light in the entire painting breaks through. These contrasts, through the complementary resources of composition and color, assemble in a single image the nymph's sterile yearning, Narcissus's fatal misunderstanding, and the echo's impotence and omnipotence.

12

FEMALE SEXUALITY AND THE ORIGIN OF SOCIETY

In the nineteenth century and even in the early twentieth, a theory in vogue among anthropologists had it that, in the early days of humanity, women had the upper hand in familial and social affairs. Various evidence of that supposed primitive matriarchy was put forward, to wit: female sculptures and the frequent figuration of female symbols in prehistoric art; a preponderant place granted to "mother goddesses" in the protohistoric period, in the Mediterranean basin and beyond; so-called primitive peoples observed in our own time, whose names and social status were passed down from the mother to her children; and, finally, many myths collected nearly everywhere in the world, all of which provide variations on a single theme. In ancient times, they say, women ruled over men. Men's subjugation lasted until they managed to seize the sacred objects—often musical instruments—from which women drew their power. Having become the sole possessors of these means for communicating with the supernatural world, the men could definitively establish their domination.

Those who granted historical verisimilitude to myths misunderstood their principal function, which is to explain why things are the way they are at present. That obliges myths to posit that things were once different. In short, myths reason in the same way as those nineteenth-century thinkers in the thrall of evolutionism, who strove to arrange in a unilinear series the institutions and customs observed in the world. Starting from the postulate that our civilization is the most complex and the most evolved, they saw the institutions of so-called primitive peoples as a reflection of those that may have existed at the beginnings of humankind. And since the Western world is governed by paternal law, they concluded that uncivilized peoples must have had, and sometimes still had, a radically different law.

The advances of ethnographic observation put an end to the illusions of matriarchy, and for a time it was possible to believe that end was definitive. We came to realize that, in a maternal legal regime as in a paternal legal regime, authority belongs to the men. The only difference is that it is exercised by the mother's brothers in one case and by her husband in the other.

Under the influence of the feminist movements and what is called "gender studies" in the United States, hypotheses of matriarchal inspiration are returning in force. But they are based on a very different, much more ambitious argument. It was in making the decisive leap from nature to culture that humanity supposedly separated itself from animality and that human societies were born. That leap would remain a mystery were it not possible to identify one or another distinctive capacity of humankind that allowed it to get off the ground. Two of these capacities were already known: the making of tools and articulate language. A third was now proposed—one, it was claimed, that was far superior. Not limited to the intellectual faculties presupposed by the first, it lay at the very heart of organic life. The first appearance of culture would no longer be a mystery but would be rooted in physiology.

Of all mammals, the human animal is the only one, according to a traditional formulation (whose importance has not been measured, however), that can make love in all seasons. Human females do not have one or several rutting seasons. Unlike other animals, they do not signal to males, by changes in coloring and the emission of odors, their periods of estrus, that is, those favorable for fertilization and gestation. And they do not reject males at other times.

We are invited to see that major difference as the factor that made possible and even determined the transition from nature to culture.

How is this thesis demonstrated? This is where things get complicated: for lack of any possible proof, the imagination enjoys free rein. Some mention the behavior of wild chimpanzees: females in heat obtain more animal-based foods from the males than do the other females. By bold extrapolation it is inferred that, when hunting became a specifically male occupation among humans, women who made themselves sexually available at all times received a larger share of the game. These women, better nourished, more robust, and as a result more fertile, were advantaged by natural selection. And there was an additional benefit: by concealing ovulation, these women would have constrained the males (in these primitive times, motivated only by the need to propagate their genes) to devote more time to them than the reproductive act by itself would have required. The women thus assured themselves lasting protection, which became increasingly useful as, over the course of evolution, the children they produced became larger and their development occurred later.

Other authors, taking the opposite view, claim that in not "advertising" (as the Americans say) their periods of estrus, women made supervision by their husbands more difficult and less effective. These men were not always the best procreators; the interest of the species, therefore, allowed women to increase their chances of being fertilized by other males.

Here, already, are two diametrically opposed interpretations of a single phenomenon: the key to monogamous marriage in one case; the remedy to its disadvantages in the other. In a highly respectable French scholarly journal (since ideas from across the Atlantic are gaining influence here as well), I found a third, no less fanciful theory, presented in all seriousness. The loss of estrus would supposedly be the origin of the prohibition of incest, which we know is practically universal in its various forms in human societies. That loss, it is claimed, and the constant availability that results, would have attracted too many men to each woman. The social order and the stability of marriage would have been compromised if every woman, via the prohibition of incest, were not made inaccessible to those who, because of a domestic life in common, were the most susceptible to temptation.

It is not explained how in very small societies the prohibition of incest would have protected women, made more desirable by the absence of estrus, from what is called a "generalized sexual commerce" with those males around them on a daily basis who were not close relatives. Above all, the proponents of that theory seem unaware of the fact that the exact opposite theory could be supported just as plausibly (or rather, implausibly).

We were told that the disappearance of estrus threatened the peace of marriages and that the prohibition of incest had to be instituted to ward off that threat. But according to other authors, it is on the contrary the existence of estrus that proved incompatible with social life. When humans began to form true societies, the ensuing danger was that every female in heat would attract all the males. The social order would not have been able to withstand it. Estrus thus had to disappear for society to come into being.

At least that last theory rests on a seductive argument. Sexual odors did not disappear entirely. In ceasing to be natural, they could become cultural. Such would be the origin of perfume, whose chemical structure even now is similar to that of organic pheromones since the ingredients composing it come from animals.

With that theory, a path opened up that some have rushed to take, once again turning the basic facts of the problem on their head. Far from positing the total loss of estrus, they assert that women could not conceal it completely because their menses, heavier than those of other mammals, often betrayed them, signaling to all that they were entering a period of fertility. Women, in competition for the males, invented a stratagem. Those who were not fertile at the time and who therefore did not attract the men's attention tried to deceive them by daubing themselves with blood or with a red pigment imitating blood. That is supposedly the origin of makeup (after that of perfume, as we have seen).

In that scenario, women are clever calculators. Another scenario denies them any talent of that kind, or rather, turns stupidity to the advantage of women who, having remained ignorant of their periods of ovulation, would have more opportunities to propagate their genes. Natural selection would favor them at the expense of more intelligent women who, understanding the link between copulation and conception, would be able to avoid copulating during estrus in order to spare themselves the difficulties of gestation.

Depending on the whims of the theory makers, the loss of estrus thus appears sometimes as an advantage, sometimes as a disadvantage. Some say that loss made it possible to strengthen marriages, others that it mitigated the biological risks of monogamous unions. It exposed humans to the social perils of promiscuity, or it prevented them. We are overcome by vertigo in the face of these contradictory, mutually annihilating interpretations. And when you can make the facts say anything at all, it is pointless to attempt to base an explanation on them.

For the last century, and in the United States itself, anthropologists have made every effort to introduce a bit of caution, seriousness, and rigor into their discipline. How could they not be saddened to see their field of study invaded, engulfed even (especially in the United States, which is quick to repudiate the old masters, but already in Great Britain, and soon, we may fear, throughout Europe), by these genital Robinson Crusoe tales? Even supposing they really took place, these revolutions, which are discussed as if they happened yesterday, date back hundreds of thousands if not millions of years. We can say nothing about such a remote past. As a result, to find a meaning for the loss of estrus, to invent a role for it that sheds light on the social life we now lead, proponents of these theories surreptitiously shift that loss to an era that, though still unknown to us, is not so distant as to prevent them from projecting its supposed effects onto the present.

It is significant that these theories about estrus developed in the United States in the wake of another theory whose aim was also to shorten time spans. According to that theory, Neanderthal man, the immediate predecessor of *Homo sapiens* (and his contemporary for a few millennia), could not have possessed articulate language because of the conformation of his larynx and pharynx. The advent of language, therefore, supposedly dates back little more than fifty thousand years.

Behind these futile attempts to ascribe simple organic causes to complicated intellectual activities, we recognize a mode of thought blinded by naturalism and empiricism. When observations that could ground a theory are lacking—which is almost always the case—that mode of thought invents them. This propensity for misrepresenting gratuitous assertions as empirical data takes us back several centuries, since it characterized anthropological thought at its beginnings.

Although the anatomical structure of Neanderthal man's throat kept him from emitting certain phonemes, it is beyond dispute that he could emit others. And phonemes of all kinds are equally suitable for differentiating meanings. The origin of language is not linked to the conformation of the speech organs. It must be sought in the neurology of the brain.

And brain neurology demonstrates that language could already have existed in remote times, long before the first appearance of *Homo sapiens* some hundred thousand years ago. Endocranial casts made from remains of *Homo habilis*, one of our distant predecessors, show that the left frontal lobe and what is called the Broca area, the seat of language, were already formed more than two million years ago. As the name given to him emphasizes, *Homo habilis* made tools, rudimentary to be sure, but corresponding to standardized forms. It is not immaterial in that respect that the component of the brain that commands the right hand is contiguous to the Broca area and that the two zones developed in concert. Nothing allows us to claim that *Homo habilis* could speak, but he had the first faculties to do so.

By contrast, there can be no doubt about *Homo erectus*, our direct predecessor, who half a million years ago carved stone tools with a careful symmetry requiring more than a dozen successive operations. It is unimaginable that these complex techniques could have been transmitted from generation to generation without instruction.

All these considerations, then, push back the first appearance of conceptual thought, articulate language, and life in society to times so remote that we cannot concoct hypotheses about them without displaying a naïveté bordering on gullibility. If we seek to place the loss of estrus at the origin of culture, we must admit that it had already occurred with *Homo erectus*, perhaps even with *Homo habilis*, species about whose physiology we know nothing except that, in terms of understanding human evolution, the really interesting things occurred in the brain, not the uterus or larynx.

To anyone who would let himself be tempted by the little estrus game, I would therefore suggest that, all in all, the least absurd hypothesis would be to place the loss of estrus in a direct relationship with the appearance of language. When women could signal their moods with words, even if they chose to express themselves in veiled terms, they no longer needed the physiological means by which they had previously made themselves understood. These old means—with their cumbersome mechanics of swelling, sweatiness, flushing, and the emission of odors—having lost their primary function and become useless, would have gradually atrophied. Culture would have shaped nature, not vice versa.

13

A LESSON IN WISDOM FROM

MAD COWS

For the Amerindians and most of the peoples who long remained without writing, mythical times were those when human beings and animals were not really distinct from one another and could communicate. These groups would have seen the decision to make historical time begin with the Tower of Babel, when humans lost the use of a common language and ceased to understand one another, as the expression of a singularly narrow view of things. The end to an original harmony, according to them, occurred on a much vaster scale; it afflicted not only humans but all living beings.

Even today we seem to remain vaguely aware of that first solidarity between all forms of life. Nothing appears more urgent to us than to instill in the minds of our young children, almost from birth, the sense of that continuity. We surround them with rubber or plush animals, and the first picture books we put before their eyes show them—well before they encounter them—the bear, the elephant, the horse, the donkey, the dog, the cat, the rooster, the hen, the mouse, the rabbit, and so on; as if it were necessary from the most tender age to make them yearn for a unity that they will quickly learn has vanished.

It is not surprising that the killing of living creatures for food poses a philosophical problem for human beings, whether or not they are conscious of it, a problem that all societies have tried to solve. The Old Testament deems it an indirect consequence of the fall. In the Garden of Eden, Adam and Eve lived on fruits and grains (Genesis 1:29). It was only with Noah that human beings became carnivorous (9:3). It is significant that this rift between humankind and the other animals immediately precedes the story of the Tower of Babel—that is, the separation of human beings from one another—as if it were the consequence or a particular case of that first rift.

This view of things makes a carnivorous diet an enrichment of sorts of the vegetarian regime. Some peoples without writing, however, see it as a barely attenuated form of cannibalism. They humanize the relationship between hunters (or fishers) and their prey by conceiving it on the model of a kinship relation, between relatives by marriage or, even more directly, between spouses (facilitated by the assimilation in all languages of the world, including our own in slang expressions, of the act of eating to that of copulation). Hunting and fishing thus look like a kind of endocannibalism.

Other peoples—and sometimes the same ones—believe that the total quantity of life existing in the universe at every moment must always be in balance. Hunters or fishers who take away a portion of life will have to reimburse it, so to speak, at the expense of their own life expectancy. That is another way of seeing the carnivorous diet as a form of cannibalism: self-cannibalism this time, since, according to that conception, one eats oneself while believing one is eating another.

About three years ago I published an article in *La Repubblica* on the so-called mad cow epidemic ("Siamo tutti cannibali," October 10–11, 1993; see chap. 9 above), which was less in the news then than it now is. In it I explained that pathologies similar to it, and to which human beings sometimes fell victim (kuru in New Guinea, new cases of Creutzfeldt-Jakob disease in Europe), were associated with practices that were properly speaking cannibalistic. Creutzfeldt-Jakob disease resulted from the administration of substances extracted from human brains to treat growth disorders. The notion of cannibalism therefore had to be broadened to include all such practices. Now we are told that the disease from the same family that is afflicting cows in several European countries, and that poses a deadly risk to the consumer, was transmitted through bone meal made from cattle and then fed to livestock. It was thus the result of the transformation of cows into cannibals by human beings, following a pattern that is not unprecedented in history. Texts contemporary to the Wars of Religion affirm that, during these bloody conflicts in France in the sixteenth century, starving Parisians were reduced to living on bread made from human bones extracted from the catacombs and ground into flour.

The link between a meat-based diet and cannibalism (a notion broadened to take on a certain universality) thus has very deep roots in thought. It has returned to prominence with the mad cow epidemic since the fear of contracting a mortal illness has been added to the horror that cannibalism, now extended to bovines, traditionally inspires in us. But having been conditioned from earliest childhood, we remain carnivores, and we fall back on substitute sources of meat. Meat consumption has dropped spectacularly, however. And how many of us, well before these events, were unable to pass a butcher's stall without feeling discomfort, seeing it already from the perspective of future centuries? Indeed, a day may come when the idea that human beings in the past raised and slaughtered living things for food and complacently displayed slabs of their flesh in shop windows will inspire the same revulsion as what travelers in the sixteenth and seventeenth centuries felt about the cannibal meals of American, Oceanian, or African indigenous peoples.

The growing vogue for animal protection movements attests to the fact that we perceive with increasing clarity the contradiction in which our customs have ensnared us, between the unity of creation as it still manifested itself when the animals entered Noah's ark and its negation by the Creator himself when they left it.

*

* *

Auguste Comte is probably one of the philosophers who paid the most attention to the problem of human beings' relationship with animals. He did so in a form that commentators have preferred to ignore, considering his discussion one of the extravagances in which the great genius often indulged. Nevertheless, it merits a moment's pause.

Comte divided animals into three categories. In the first are those that, in one way or another, pose a danger for human beings. He proposed quite simply destroying them.

He placed in a second category the species protected and raised by humans for food: cattle, pigs, sheep, barnyard animals. Over the millennia, he writes, human beings have so profoundly transformed these species that they cannot even be called animals anymore. They must be seen as "nutrient laboratories," where the organic compounds necessary for our subsistence are developed.

Even as Comte excludes that second category from animality, he integrates the third into the human race. It comprises the sociable species that provide us with companions and often even serve as active assistants, animals whose "mental inferiority has been greatly exaggerated." Some, such as dogs and cats, are carnivorous. Others, because they are herbivores, do not have an intellectual level high enough to make them serviceable. Comte recommends turning them into carnivores. He does not consider that impossible because in Norway, when there is no fodder, cattle are fed dried fish. Certain herbivores could thus attain the highest degree of perfection that animal nature can entail. More active and more intelligent as a result of their new diet, they would be more amenable to devoting themselves to their masters, conducting themselves as servants of humanity. They could assume the primary responsibility for watching over energy sources, and machines could be entrusted to them, which would free up humans for other tasks. Comte acknowledges that his vision is utopian, but no more so than the idea of the transmutation of metals, which, after all, is the origin of modern chemistry. The application of the idea of transmutation to animals only extends the utopian ideal from the material order to the order of biology.

These views, a century and half old, are prophetic in several respects, paradoxical in others. It is only too true that, directly or indirectly, human beings are causing the disappearance of countless species and that others are gravely threatened. We need only think of bears, wolves, tigers, rhinoceroses, elephants, whales, and so on, plus the species of insects and other invertebrates being destroyed day by day by the deterioration of the natural environment caused by humans.

Also prophetic, and to an extent Comte could not have imagined, is his vision of the animals that human beings make their food, creatures mercilessly reduced to the condition of nutrient laboratories. Factory farming of calves, pigs, and chickens provides the most horrible illustration of this process. Even the European Parliament has recently become disturbed by it.

Equally prophetic is the idea that the animals constituting the third category conceived by Comte could become human beings' active collaborators. This is attested by the increasingly diverse missions entrusted to guide dogs, the use of specially trained monkeys to assist the seriously disabled, and the hopes raised by work with dolphins.

Even the transmutation of herbivores into carnivores is prophetic, as the tragedy of mad cow disease proves. In this case, however, things did not come about as Comte anticipated. We have turned herbivores into carnivores, but that transformation may not be as fundamental as we believe. Some have argued that ruminants are not true herbivores because they feed primarily on microorganisms, which in turn feed on plant matter fermented in the ruminant's specially adapted stomach.

Above all, that transformation did not benefit human beings' active assistants but rather occurred at the expense of the animals Comte calls "nutrient laboratories," a fatal error that he himself had warned against. "An excess of animality," he said, "would be harmful to them." Harmful to them and also to us: Is it not by conferring on them an excess of animality (through their transformation into cannibals and not only into carnivores) that we have, unintentionally to be sure, changed our "nutrient laboratories" into death laboratories?

* *

Mad cow disease has not yet reached every country. Italy, I believe, has remained free of it so far. Perhaps the disease will be forgotten soon: the epidemic may die out on its own, as the British scientists predict; or vaccines or treatments may be discovered; or a rigorous policy may guarantee the health of the animals intended for slaughter. But other scenarios are also conceivable.

Some suspect that, contrary to received ideas, the disease could cross the species barrier. Striking all the animals we use for food, it could settle in for a long time and take its place among the evils arising from industrial civilization, which with increasing gravity interfere with the satisfaction of all living beings' needs.

Already we breathe only polluted air. Water, also polluted, is no longer a resource believed to be limitless: we know it is rationed both in agriculture and in domestic use. Since the appearance of AIDS, sexual relations have entailed a fatal risk. All these phenomena cause upheaval in humankind's living conditions and will continue to do so, ushering in a new era. The mortal danger now represented by a meat-based diet would simply fall in line with all the others.

That is not the only factor that could compel human beings to turn away from meat. In a world where the global human population will probably have doubled in less than a century, cattle and other livestock are becoming formidable competitors. It has been calculated that in the United States two-thirds of the grain produced is fed to livestock. And let us not forget that these animals yield many fewer calories in the form of meat than they consumed over the course of their lives (only a fifth, I've been told, in the case of a chicken). An expanding human population will soon need the current grain production as a whole to survive; nothing will remain for cattle and barnyard animals. All humans will therefore have to model their diet on that of India and China, where animal flesh fulfills only a very small portion of protein and calorie needs. We may even have to give up meat completely since, as the population has increased, the surface area of cultivable lands has decreased as a result of erosion and urbanization. In addition, oil and gas reserves are dropping, and water resources are drying up. Conversely, experts estimate that, if humanity were to become fully vegetarian, the areas now cultivated could feed twice the current population.

It is noteworthy that in Western societies the consumption of meat is tending to fall off on its own. Apparently, we are beginning to change our diet. If so, the mad cow epidemic, by turning consumers away from meat, would only be accelerating a development already under way. It would add only a mystical component, the vague feeling that our species is paying the price for having violated the natural order.

Agronomists will take on the task of increasing the protein content of food plants, chemists of producing synthetic proteins in industrial quantities. But even if spongiform encephalopathy (the scientific name for mad cow disease and other related ailments) settles in for the duration, chances are that the appetite for meat will not disappear. The satisfaction of that appetite will simply become a rare, costly, and risky occasion. (Japan has something similar with *fugu*, the pufferfish, which has an exquisite flavor, it is said, but if improperly eviscerated can be a lethal poison.) Meat will appear on the menu only under extraordinary circumstances. It will be consumed with the same mix of pious reverence and anxiety that, according to ancient travelers, accompanied the cannibal meals of certain peoples. In both cases, it is a matter of communing with ancestors and of incorporating into ourselves—at our own risk and peril—the dangerous substance of living beings that were or have become enemies.

Livestock breeding, having become unprofitable, will completely disappear; meat, purchased in high-end luxury boutiques, will come only from hunting. Our former herds, left to their own devices, will be only one kind of game among others in rural areas that have returned to the wild.

It cannot therefore be asserted that the expansion of a civilization that aspires to be global will standardize the planet. Populations that were formerly better distributed will cram into megalopolises as big as provinces (as we are already seeing), evacuating other areas. Permanently deserted by their inhabitants, these areas might return to archaic conditions; here and there, the strangest forms of life could make a place for themselves. Instead of heading toward monotony, the evolution of humanity may accentuate contrasts, even create new ones, reestablishing the reign of diversity. Such is the lesson in wisdom that, in breaking millennial habits, we may someday have learned from mad cows.

14

THE RETURN OF THE
MATERNAL UNCLE

The industrial or military applications of modern physics and chemistry have acquainted us with the notions of critical mass and critical temperature. They concern thresholds below or above which matter manifests properties that remain hidden under ordinary conditions. One might have believed these properties nonexistent, even inconceivable, before the thresholds were crossed.

Human societies too have their critical points, which they reach when the course of their existence is seriously disrupted. Suddenly, latent properties reveal themselves: sometimes they are vestiges of an ancient state that resurfaces after it was believed to have disappeared; sometimes they are still present but normally invisible, buried in the deepest part of the social structure. Often, in fact, they are both at once.

I was reflecting on these matters a few months ago while reading in the press the text of Earl Spencer's speech at the funeral of his sister, Princess Diana. Most unexpectedly, his remarks revived the role of the maternal uncle. Some may have believed that, in the present state of society, this is merely one kinship relation among others to which no particular significance is attached. By contrast, in our society's past and in the present of many exotic societies, the mother's brother was or remains a key player in the familial and social structure. It seems quite a coincidence that Earl Spencer lives in South Africa, since a famous article by Radcliffe-Brown appeared in the *South African Journal of Science* in 1924 bearing this title: "The Mother's Brother in South Africa." In it the author sheds light on the importance of that role. He was one of the first to seek to understand what its significance might be.

In the first place Earl Spencer, in imputing his sister's misfortunes to her ex-husband and to the royal family as a whole, assumed the position of "wife-giver," to use the jargon of ethnologists, who retains a right of access to his sister or daughter and can intervene if either he or she believes she is being mistreated. Above all, he affirms that between him and his nephews, his sister's sons, a special bond exists that gives him the right and the duty to protect them from their father and the paternal lineage.

Such a structural role allotted to the maternal uncle is not recognized by contemporary society. It was so recognized in the Middle Ages, however, and may also have been in antiquity. In Greek, "uncle" is *theîos* (from which the Italian, Spanish, and Portuguese terms *zío* and *tío* are derived), which is to say, "divine relation," which would suggest that this relative held a place of choice in the family constellation. That place was so important in the Middle Ages that the plot of most of the chansons de geste turns on the relationship between the maternal uncle and his nephew(s). Roland is the uterine nephew of Charlemagne; Vivien, of William of Orange; Gautier, of Raoul de Cambrai; Perceval, of the Grail King; Gawain, of King Arthur; Tristan, of King Mark; Gamwell, of Robin Hood; and on and on. That kinship created bonds so strong that they overshadowed all others: *The Song of Roland* does not even mention the hero's father.

The maternal uncle and the nephew assisted each other. The nephew received presents from his uncle; the uncle knighted him and sometimes even supplied him with a wife. The intensity of the feelings between them is expressed eloquently in the words attributed to Charlemagne in another chanson de geste, *L'entrée en Espagne* (*Entry into Spain*), when Roland leaves him to go into battle: "If I lose you / moaned the emperor, I will be all alone / Like a poor lady when she has lost her man."

*
* *

The relationship between uncle and nephew, it seems, is less apparent in Italian and Spanish chansons de geste than in French and Germanic ones. Perhaps that is because in the Germanic tradition it is situated within a larger institutional framework, called "fosterage" in English. The custom of fosterage, strictly observed in Ireland and Scotland, stipulated that the children of noble lineages be entrusted to another family, who reared them and saw to it that they were educated. As a result, the moral and sentimental bonds between these parties were stronger than those acknowledged within their birth families. The same custom also existed in continental Europe, at least in the form of so-called uncle fosterage. The noble child was entrusted to his mother's family, generally represented by the maternal uncle, for whom the child occupied the position of *nourri* (literally, "nurtured one"), which he would thereafter retain. In Old French, the word *nourri* had a sense much broader than simply that of being fed.

These practices were once taken as evidence of an ancient predominance of maternal law and matrilineal filiation, which, however, is nowhere attested in ancient Europe. We now understand that, on the contrary, they are one effect among others of patrilineal filiation. It is precisely because the father holds familial authority that the maternal uncle, a true "male mother," assumes the countervailing role. In a society of matrilineal filiation, conversely, the maternal uncle exerts familial authority and is feared and obeyed by his nephew. A correlation thus exists between the attitude toward the maternal uncle and that toward the father. In societies where the relationship between father and son is casual, that between uncle and nephew is strict; and where the father appears as the austere agent of familial authority, the uncle is treated with tenderness and liberty.

Countless societies throughout the world illustrate one or the other arrangement: filiation is transmitted either directly through the men, from father to son, or through the intermediary of women, from uncle to nephew. In both cases, the maternal uncle is part of a four-term system (along with his sister, her husband, and the children born of their union) that unites in the most economical way conceivable the three types of family relations necessary for a kinship structure to exist, namely, a relation of consanguinity, a relation of alliance, and a relation of filiation: in other words, a brother–sister relationship, a husband–wife relationship, and a parents–children relationship.

That structure has become nearly invisible, submerged in the complexity of modern societies, but it acquired new relevancy through Earl Spencer's remarks. He defined flawlessly the internal relationships within a four-term familial system. His sister and he, he said, were united by a warmth and closeness dating back to their earliest childhood: "We spent such an enormous amount of time together—the two youngest in the family."[1] Conversely, the relationship between the princess and her husband and his lineage was marked by "anguish . . . tearful despair." And just as the relationship between brother and sister stands opposed to that between husband and wife, so too, in the earl's speech, the relationship between uncle and nephews, to whom he pledges to give a kinder upbringing, [contrasts to that between father and sons.] That is, two sets of contrasting relationships, one positive, the other negative, correspond exactly within a structure that can rightly be considered the kinship atom since it is impossible to conceive of one more simple (though there are more complicated ones).

*
* *

Contrary to what has long been believed, consanguinity is not the foundation of the family. Because of the prohibition of incest, which is practically universal though realized in many different forms, a man can obtain a woman only from another man, who gives his daughter or sister away. There is thus no need to explain how the maternal uncle makes his appearance within the kinship structure. He does not make an appearance, he is its condition, an immediate given within it.

That structure, still recognizable two or three centuries ago, disintegrated under the influence of the demographic, social, economic, and political changes that accompanied the industrial revolution, sometimes as causes, sometimes as effects. For us, unlike what occurs in societies without writing, kinship ties no longer exert a regulatory role over all social relations; the overall coherence of these relations depends on other factors.

The intense emotion stirred throughout the world by the death of Princess Diana is explained in great part by the fact that this tragedy placed her at the crossroads of major themes in folklore (the king's son who marries a shepherdess, the evil stepmother) and religious themes (the sinner put to death who, by her sacrifice, takes on the sins of the newly converted). It is then easier to understand how the tragedy allowed other archaic structures to reappear. A maternal uncle was able to embrace a role that, in the past of our own societies, would have belonged to him and that still belongs to him in others, even though that role now lacks any legal or even customary foundation. "We, your blood family," proclaims Earl Spencer, as if the rights over his nephews that he claims for himself had a basis in mores. "She would want us today to pledge ourselves to protecting her beloved boys William and Harry from a similar fate and I do this here Diana on your behalf . . . to continue the imaginative way in which you were steering these two exceptional young men." In the name of what authority could he aspire to do so without resuscitating a kinship structure that used to predominate in human societies, that was believed to have disappeared from our own, and that, as a result of a crisis, has risen again to the actors' consciousness?

*
* *

The work of a young Chinese ethnologist trained in France has just introduced new documents regarding the preeminent place granted to the maternal uncle in certain exotic societies. An ethnic group along the border of China in the Himalayas possesses a familial and social system that is remarkable in every respect. Back in the thirteenth century, it sparked Marco Polo's curiosity. The domestic cell—which we hardly dare call a family, so far removed is it from our usual notions—is composed of a brother, a sister, and her children. These children, who belong exclusively to the maternal lineage, are the fruit of sexual relations the woman is permitted to have with any man to whom she is not related (since the prohibition of incest applies here as elsewhere). These unions, though sometimes relatively long-lasting, are usually confined to furtive, short-lived visits. The woman may receive an unlimited number of these visits, to which the men dedicate themselves as soon as night has fallen. When a child is born, there is no way of knowing which of these occasional lovers is the father, and in fact, no one cares to know. The kinship terminology does not include any term to which the sense of "father" or "husband" could be attached.[2]

The author of these interesting observations believes, rather naively, that he has discovered a unique case that overturns all received ideas about the family, kinship, and marriage. That is a mistake in two respects. The Na represent a case, perhaps an extreme case, of a system for which other examples have long been known, especially in Nepal, southern India, and Africa. And such cases, far from demolishing received ideas, illustrate a familial structure that is simply a symmetrical and inverted image of our own.

These societies obliterate the category of husband, just as we ourselves have obliterated the category of maternal uncle (for which our kinship terminologies no longer have a distinct word). Not, of course, that in one or another of our families that uncle cannot occasionally play a role, but that role is not written into the system in advance. There is thus nothing surprising about a family that has no role for the husband; or at least, it is no more surprising than a family without a role anticipated for the maternal uncle, which seems natural to us. No one would claim that our own societies invalidate kinship and marriage theories. Nor does Na society. These are quite simply societies that do not grant, or no longer grant, a regulatory value to kinship and marriage but rather turn to other mechanisms to assure their functioning. Kinship and marriage systems do not possess the same importance in all cultures. In some, they provide the active principle that regulates social relations. In others, such as our own and no doubt that of the Na as well, that function is absent or very diminished.

The point of these reflections, which began with an event that a few months ago stunned the public imagination, is this: to better understand certain driving forces in the operation of societies, we cannot make use only of those that are the most remote from us in time or space.

For interpretations of ancient or recent customs whose meaning was no longer known, people used to turn almost automatically to ethnology, which viewed them as survivals or vestiges of a social state still present among "uncivilized" peoples. Contrary to that outmoded primitivism, we have come to realize that forms of social life and types of organization well attested in our history can in some circumstances become current once again and can cast a retrospective light on societies very remote from us in space or time. Between so-called complex or evolved societies and those wrongly called primitive or archaic, the distance is less great than some may have believed. The faraway illuminates the near, but the near can also illuminate the faraway.

15

PROOF BY NEW MYTH

The proponents of structural analysis know they are vulnerable to a criticism to which they really must respond from time to time. They are reproached for what is seen as an inherent weakness in their project: they misuse analogy by confining themselves to the most superficial ones, or they use all means available, resorting to heterogeneous and therefore questionable analogies. For some, the limitless series of associations produced by structural analysis resembles a game in favor among schoolchildren, which consists of exchanging words, each of which begins with the syllable or syllables ending the previous word, while drawing from the most incongruous sectors of the lexicon.

The appeal of that game for young minds would merit consideration. It cannot be explained as a search for assonances that would simply be poetic. Assonance is one of the resources poetry uses to gain access to realities inexpressible in prose. In fact, that game evokes in rudimentary form a versification process with which the old poets were familiar, the use of what were called chained, concatenated, appended, or fraternized rhymes. It also brings to mind the "pivot words," *kakekotoba*, in Japanese versification, in which a single syllable or single group of syllables takes on two meanings simultaneously. Rhyme, which also plays on similarity and difference, highlights relationships of equivalence between sound and meaning: "It would be an unsound oversimplification to treat rhyme merely from the standpoint of sound. Rhyme necessarily involves a semantic relationship" (Jakobson 1960, 14).

You will therefore not get rid of the chains of analogies of structural analysis by relegating them to the subordinate place that, in a different genre, would similarly be misassigned to rhymes, since both are more meaningful than you might imagine. The grounding for these analogies is that, as the terms of a hypothetico-deductive reasoning, they lead to conclusions for which it must be possible to provide the proof. I would like to demonstrate this with an example (Lévi-Strauss 1985).

Let pottery clay serve as our starting point. From there, we move on to Nightjar because, in certain myths, clay is the effect of Nightjar and Nightjar is the cause of clay. The image of Nightjar, as soon as it is formed, reverses into that of Sloth; by virtue of several traits, these two form a pair of opposites. The similarity of Sloth's way of life to that of other animals then leads to their all being subsumed under the concept of arboreal fauna, which leads to the tribe of dwarfs with no anus, a figural representation of that fauna; and from there, to dwarfs with no mouth, through a relation of inverted symmetry that occurs with a change in hemisphere.

These successive transfers, sometimes logical, sometimes rhetorical or even geographical, are based on relations of contiguity, resemblance, equivalence, or inversion. They are syllepses, metonomies, or metaphors. How are we to convince readers that these choices are not arbitrary, designed for the needs of the cause on an ad hoc basis? Do they not move us further and further away from the starting point, as if along the way we had forgotten pottery, whose mythic status provided the inquiry with its raison d'être? One critic, after recalling the thesis that arboreal fauna may be conceived in American mythology as the transformation of a tribe of dwarfs, objects: "But that is only supposition, since . . . most of these relationships are merely postulated, without any myths being put forward to justify them. . . . Considering the strategic place these myths would have to occupy in *The Jealous Potter* in terms of providing proof, that cannot fail to be significant" (Abad Márquez 1995, 336).

Yet that circuitous route, on which new postulates and new hypotheses appear at every turn, happens to be immediately and universally validated when a previously unknown myth surfaces that short-circuits the intermediaries and unites the conclusion and the premises. Such is the case for a myth of the Tatuyo Indians from the Vaupés region, collected by Elsa Gómez-Imbert, who, aware of its importance for my argument, communicated it to me before publishing it. I would like to express my thanks to her here.

The myth can be divided into two parts. The second, which I leave aside temporarily, deals with the fabrication of pots, a female occupation, and explains why it became laborious. The first part dates back further in time, to the origin of clay, the raw material for pottery.

An Indian who was out fishing came upon the Forest Spirit, No-Anus. The Indian farted in his presence. The Spirit, astonished, asked to know the origin of the noise. The man explained that his anus was speaking. The Spirit admitted he had no anus. The Indian proposed to make one for him and drove a sharpened wooden rod into the Sprit's behind with such violence that the Spirit died as a result. From that hole clay is now extracted, the rotted flesh of the Spirit (Gómez-Imbert 1990).

A complex argument extending over a hundred pages was required to demonstrate that the myths on the origin of clay and those on dwarfs with no anus belong to the same series, and then to determine the reasons this is so. The validity of that long trajectory is now proven by a myth that identifies No-Anus with clay.

*
* *

In the same way, a myth that remained outside the field of inquiry allows us to shed light on a connection that, in this case, I was constrained to postulate between two sets of myths: one on the origin of pottery, the other on the origin of the colors of birds.

I begin by noting that, in the Americas, myths on the origin of pottery are divided into two subsets, one dealing with the origin of pottery, the other—like the second part of the Tatuyo myth—with the fabrication of decorations on pots. That art was taught to women by the supernatural mistress of pottery, whom the myths also represent in the form of the rainbow, a monstrous serpent living at the bottom of the waters. The polychrome motifs adorning the serpent's skin were copied by the potters, and even today these motifs inspire the decoration of their works.

But other myths depict that serpent in a very different story. Birds, the enemy of the serpent, got together to destroy it. After killing the monster, they divided up its remains and, depending on the piece of skin that fell to each bird (representative of a species), each acquired its distinctive plumage.

By means of polychromy, a connection is thus established between the colors of birds, decorated pottery, and clay. At first sight, nothing makes that connection necessary. Nevertheless, one myth allows us to demonstrate the unity of the two series. It comes from the Maya Indians of the Yucatan. Granted, that is a long way from the Amazon, but after all, our first reflections on the role of polychromy in South American myths led us to Mexico (Lévi-Strauss 1964, 329; 1967, 26).

Several versions of this myth are known to us. According to the most recent, the birds, who quarreled constantly among themselves, were summoned to an assembly by the Great Ancestor to name a king. Wild Turkey proposed himself as a candidate, pointing out his well-proportioned size and his melodious voice—but his feathers were not beautiful enough. He borrowed those of Nightjar and was chosen. Meanwhile Nightjar waited in vain for the favors Turkey had promised him in return. The birds found him hiding in the woods, stripped bare, half dead from the cold. Overcome with pity, each one gave him one of its feathers. That is why today Nightjar has a motley plumage (Boccara 1966, 97). It is true that Nightjar has a plumage in shades of gray, fawn, brown, and black. Its dark and understated hues blend into the color of the ground or of the tree on which these birds squat.

The myth obviously follows a regressive course. Contrary to the myths that recount how birds acquired their distinctive plumage, this one tells how Nightjar lost his and fell back into chromatic indistinction, which was originally the lot of all birds. The approach taken by the myths in the alternate series, the one on the origin of pottery, is the same: they tell how an indiscreet woman (guilty, that is, of oral incontinence) lost the pots received from her supernatural benefactress. They broke into pieces, which turned back into balls of clay, a material identified in the Tatuyo myth with a person afflicted with anal retention (instead of being too open above, he is too closed below).

The path leading back from decorated pottery to clay and the one leading back from the colored plumage of birds to the motley and drab plumage of Nightjar are thus parallel; or, if one prefers, where color is concerned, Nightjar is to the other birds what clay is to decorated pottery. Thus the choice of the Jivaro myths (which combine Nightjar and clay) as a generative cell for the mythology of pottery is validated.

When compared to the long chains of associations that had to be laid out from one myth to another to arrive at a demonstration, the myth serving as proof displays the characteristic of a residue: only the essential remains. As in arithmetic, the proof consists of replacing a complicated operation (in this case, the one that unfolded by means of numerous myths) with a simpler, equivalent operation performed on a single myth, then of verifying that the two results coincide.

But even if the proof provides an accurate result, nothing as yet assures us that it was not obtained by chance or that the links correspond to something real outside the analyst's mind. To reach that point, one would have to multiply the number of proofs. The comparison with arithmetic is risky; all we can take from it is the warning to be cautious. The mathematical proof known as "casting out nines" (*preuve par neuf*) has something in common with the proof by a myth described as new (*preuve par mythe qualifié de neuf*) either because it was unknown at the time of the inquiry or because it had not been encountered along the way: namely, it is only plausible and can at most lay claim to a good probability. But that is already a great deal, especially in what are known as the human sciences.

Bibliography

Abad, Márquez, L. V. 1995. *La Mirada distante sobre Lévi-Strauss*. Madrid: Siglo veintiuno de España Editores.

Boccara M. 1996. "Puhuy, l'amoureux déçu: La mythologie de l'Engoulevent en pays Maya." *Journal d'agriculture traditionnelle et de botanique appliquée* 38, no. 2: 95–109.

Gómez-Imbert, E. 1990. "La façon des poteries: Mythe sur l'origine de la poterie." *Amerindia* 15: 193–227.

Jakobson, R. 1960. "Linguistics and Poetics." In *Style in Language*, ed. Thomas A. Sebeok. Cambridge, Mass.: MIT Press.

Lévi-Strauss, C. 1964. *Le cru et le cuit*. Paris: Plon.

———. 1967. *Du miel aux cendres*. Paris: Plon.

———. 1985. *La potière jalouse*. Paris: Plon.

16

CORSI E RICORSI: IN VICO'S WAKE

I recently encountered a theory put forward by an American professor of medicine, who writes that the proliferation of the human race can be likened to a cancer on the planet. The rigor and technical precision of his demonstration are impressive. My own incompetence does not allow me to offer anything more than a simplified version.

At the beginning of the Quaternary period in Africa, he explains, stem cells originating in a line of land vertebrates, and more specifically in primates, produced humanoid tissues. Healthy so long as they remained where they were, they became a malignancy in the Near East through dermic contact with richer and more diversified foodstuffs. They then became out-and-out tumors following the absorption of plant and animal tissues obtained through domestication.

These malignant cells migrated in the form of agricultural microsatellites into submucous regions of southern Europe and Asia. Metastases developed in the Near East itself, appearing as thick "urbanoid" patches that displayed numerous lithic inclusions followed by cuprous and ferrous inclusions.

Long confined to the eastern hemisphere, these aggregate tumors triggered the malignancy, perhaps already latent, of similar cells in the western hemisphere. That phenomenon, known by the name "Columbian progression," produced Hispanic and Anglo-Saxon clones through cellular recombinations.

As it worsened, the disease manifested itself as a generalized feverish state and acute respiratory distress prompted by cultural factors: the inhalation of oil distillates, a diminution of the overall quantity of oxygen, the formation of cavities in the forest lungs. The preterminal phase was indicated by elevated levels of toxic metabolites in the blood, abnormal rates of foreign chemical bodies coming from organic insecticides and from oil slicks on the surface of the oceans, and embolisms of metallic and plastic materials. A declining vascularization caused the necrosis of tumor growths, primarily those dating back several centuries, with a cell count surpassing six billion. Their urban nuclei burst from within and collapsed, leaving only endotoxic and sterile cysts behind them.[1]

Such would be the diagnosis and prognosis that a physician from beyond earth might make of our planet, perceived globally as an ecosystem. But even if the preceding portrait were viewed only as an ingenious metaphor, it would be rich in lessons: namely, that the same language can describe, and in detail, living phenomena belonging either to individual or to collective history.

We thereby gain a better understanding of the two existing types of explanation. One moves backward from the consequent to the antecedent and seeks to determine the cause or series of causes from which the phenomenon results. The other follows an approach that is transversal in some sense: it sees the phenomenon to be explained as the transposition of a model that, on another level, possesses the same structure and the same properties. It therefore constitutes a sufficient reason for the first phenomenon. The problem of the origin of language provides another, no less revealing example of such relationships.

Research under way for the last fifty years or so proves that certain properties of articulate language are not beyond the reach of a few species of primates. Nevertheless, human language is distinguished from all messages emitted by animals in their natural environment. What is proper to articulate language is, first, the power of the imagination and of creativity; and second, the ability to deal with abstractions and with objects and facts distant in space and time. Finally and above all, the absolutely original character of human language consists in its dual articulation: a first level is composed of purely distinctive units that, at a second level, combine to form significant units consisting of words and sentences.

We do not know what organic preconditions may have led to that universal cerebral capacity in our species. In the absence of a biological theory of the origin of language, the refusal in the past on the part of the Société Linguistique de Paris to allow any debate on the theme remains valid. We have no means of knowing how human language was gradually able to develop from animal communication. The difference between them is one of nature, not of degree. In fact, the problem has always appeared so insoluble that the ancients—and even a few moderns—made human language a divine institution.

The discovery of the genetic code rendered these speculations obsolete. It revealed that, at a level very remote from human language but underlying it (since it too is a manifestation of life), a model consistent with articulate language exists. The verbal code and the genetic code—and they alone—operate by means of a finite number of discrete units, meaningless as phonemes, that combine to produce minimal signifying units comparable to words. These words form sentences that even have punctuation marks, and a syntax governs these molecular messages. That is not all: as in human language, the words of the genetic code can change meaning as a function of the context. And though the role of learning in the acquisition of language must not be underestimated, the aptitude of human beings to master linguistic structures in their early years must necessarily stem from instructions coded in their germ cells. The question of genetic inheritance arises as soon as the foundation of human language is at issue. The isomorphism observed between the structure of the genetic code and the structure underlying all the verbal codes of human languages goes far beyond mere metaphor. It invites us to conceive of that universal architectonics as a molecular inheritance of Homo sapiens (and already of Homo erectus, if not even Homo habilis, in whom, it seems, the cerebral gyri on which the use of language depends were already present). Linguistic structures would thus be modeled on the structural principles of communication as it functions at the molecular level. In the same way, the proliferation of the human race, transposed to the cellular level, appeared to us to be modeled on the nosography of cancer.

Let us now consider a third problem, that of the origin of life in society, which philosophers since antiquity have never ceased to ponder. The difficulty is the same as that regarding the origin of language: between the absence and the presence of articulate language, the division is so sharp that all efforts to identify intermediate forms are futile. And yet forms of that transition exist, provided we seek them at deeper levels: the cellular level for demographic expansion, the molecular level for language, and the cellular again for sociability.

The transition from solitary life to life in society is directly observable and scientifically explicable in one species of terrestrial amoebae. These single-celled creatures lead an independent existence without any contact with their congeners, so long as the food available is sufficient. But if a food shortage should arise, the amoebae begin to secrete a substance that attracts them to one another. They form a mass and turn into an organism of a new type with diversified functions. In this social phase, they move as a body toward warmer and more humid zones where food is plentiful, after which the society disintegrates, the individuals disperse, and each resumes its separate life.

What is remarkable about these observations is that the substance produced by the amoebae, by means of which they attract one another and form into a multicellular social creature, is none other than a well-known chemical substance, cyclical adenosine monophosphate, which governs the communication between the cells of multicellular beings (like ourselves) and thus makes each individual body an enormous society. And that same substance is secreted by the bacteria that the amoebae feed on: the amoebae find the bacteria by perceiving the chemical. In other words, the substance that attracts predators to their prey is the same one that attracts predators to one another and forms them into a society.

At that humble level of cellular life, the contradiction encountered by Hobbes, and before him by Bacon—and by so many philosophers in their wake—thus finds its solution. They sought to resolve the antinomy between two maxims held to be equally true: that man is a wolf to man and that man is also a god to man, *homo homini lupus, homo homini deus.* The antinomy disappears as soon as it is acknowledged that the difference between the two states is only a matter of degree.

Terrestrial amoebae, taken as models, lead us to conceive of social life as a state in which individuals attract one another just enough to bring them closer together but not so much that, pressures having mounted, they would end up destroying one another or even devouring one another. Sociability thus appears as the lower limit, the benign modality so to speak, of aggressiveness. The daily life of human societies—our own is no exception—and the major crises they go through, would provide many arguments in support of that interpretation.

The three examples I have chosen place the problems of origin in a completely different light than is usually shed on them. These problems remain insoluble so long as one aspires to go back to the causes since in prior states certain essential properties of the phenomenon we would like to explain are always missing. The obstructed horizon is cleared and the question of genesis ceases to arise when we discover somewhere another entity on which the one we are seeking to understand is patterned. We no longer have to wonder how it came to be since it was already there.

That perspective is not new. Medieval thinkers had a notion of it, and it can be found in the eighteenth century in Vico's theory of *corsi e ricorsi*, according to which every period of human history replicates the model of a period corresponding to it in a previous cycle. These periods are in a relation of formal homology. The parallelism between the ancients and the moderns, which Vico takes as an example, proves that the entire history of human societies repeats eternally certain typical situations. Is that not what our three examples—if we give them some credit—also illustrate? In terms of the collectivity, demographic expansion appeared to us to be a *ricorso* of cancerous growth, the linguistic code a *ricorso* of the genetic code, and the sociability of multicellular creatures a *ricorso* of sociability visible at the unicellular level.

No doubt Vico restricted his theory to the history of human societies as it unfolded over time. But for him, beyond the empirical data, it was primarily the means to achieve "an ideal eternal history traversed in time by the histories of all nations."[2] Granted, his project initially relied on a distinction between the world of nature—known to God alone, since he made it—and the human or civic world made by human beings, which they can therefore know. Nevertheless, that curvature of human history, which obliges it to turn back perpetually on itself, is an effect, affirms Vico, of the will of divine providence. When, through the theory of *corsi e ricorsi* human beings become aware of that law to which their history is subject, a corner of the veil is lifted. Through the back door, so to speak, they have access to that will and are able to recognize it at work on a much vaster stage, in this case the one constituted by all the living phenomena of which human history is a part.

Hence, the theory of *corsi e ricorsi*, sometimes considered an inconsequential oddity in Vico's body of work, may in fact have considerable import. If, in fact, human beings' consciousness of their own history reveals that divine providence acts by always reusing the same models, finite in number, it becomes possible to extrapolate from the particular will of providence vis-à-vis human beings to its general will. Although the state of science in Vico's time did not yet allow him to move in that direction, his theory opens a path to knowledge leading from the structure of thought to the structure of reality.

NOTES

Santa Claus Burned as Heretic

Published originally as "Le Père Noël supplicié," *Les Temps modernes* 77 (1952): 1572–90.

1. [In the French tradition, Père Fouettard (Father Flog) accompanies Père Noël (Santa Claus or Father Christmas) on his rounds, dispensing coal and floggings to naughty children—trans.]

2. Quoted in J. Brand, *Observations on Popular Antiquities*, new ed. (London, 1900), 243.

3. On this point, see A. Varagnac, *Civilisation traditionnelle et genre de vie* (Paris, 1948), 92, 122 and passim.

4. S. Reinach, "L'origine des prières pour les morts," in *Cultes, mythes, religions* (Paris, 1905), 1:319.

1. "Topsy-Turvydom"

Originally published as "Se il mondo è alla rovescia," *La Repubblica*, August 7, 1989.

2. Is There Only One Type of Development?

Originally published in two parts: "Mercanti in fiera," *La Repubblica*, November 13, 1990; "Contadino chissà perchè," *La Repubblica*, November 14, 1990.

3. Social Problems:
Ritual Female Excision and Medically Assisted Reproduction

Originally published as "Il segreto delle donne," *La Repubblica*, November 14, 1989.

4. Presentation of a Book by Its Author

Originally published as "Gli uomini della nebbia e del vento," *La Repubblica*, September 10, 1991.

5. The Ethnologist's Jewels

Originally published as "Ma perchè ci mettano i gioielli?" *La Repubblica*, May 21, 1991.

1. D'Arcy Wentworth Thompson, *On Growth and Form* (Cambridge: Cambridge University Press, 1917; 2nd ed., 1952).
2. *Le trésor de Saint-Dénis*, Louvre Museum, until June 17, 1991.
3. Karl Marx, "The Precious Metals," chap. 2, part 4 in *A Contribution to the Critique of Political Economy*, trans. S. W. Ryazanskaya (Moscow: Progress Publishers, 1859; reprint, Marxists.org, 1993), http://www.marxists.org/archive/marx/works/download/Marx_Contribution_to_the_Critique_of_Political_Economy.pdf.

6. Portraits of Artists

Originally published as "La statua che divenne madre," *La Repubblica*, February 23, 1992.

1. J. R. Walker, *Lakota Belief and Ritual* (Lincoln: University of Nebraska Press, 1991), 165–66.

2. F. Boas, *Tsimshian Mythology* (Washington, DC: Government Printing Office, 1916), 555.

3. M. Séguin, ed., *The Tsimshian: Images of the Past, Views of the Present* (Vancouver: University of British Columbia), 164.

4. F. Boas, "The Nass River Indians," *Report of the British Association for the Advancement of Science for 1895*, 580.

5. Séguin, *The Tsimshian*, 287–88.

6. J. R. Swanton, *Haïda Texts: Memoirs of the American Museum of National History* 14 (1908): 457–89.

7. J. R. Swanton, *Tlingit Myths and Texts* (Washington, DC: Government Printing Office, 1909), 181–82.

8. Boas, *Tsimshian Mythology*, 152–54.

7. Montaigne and America

Originally published as "Come Montaigne scopri l'America," *La Repubblica*, September 11, 1992.

8. Mythic Thought and Scientific Thought

Originally published as "L'Ultimo degli Irochesi," *La Repubblica*, February 7, 1993.

1. Giambattista Vico, *The New Science of Giambattista Vico,* trans. from the 3rd ed. (1744) by Thomas Goddard Bergin and Max Harold Fisch (Ithaca, NY: Cornell University Press, 1948), book 2, sec. 2, chap. 2.5, para. 409, p. 118, https://archive.org/stream/newscience ofgiam030174mbp/newscienceofgiam030174mbp_djvu.txt. For the following quotation, see the same paragraph.

9. We Are All Cannibals

Originally published as "Siamo tutti cannibali," *La Repubblica*, October 10, 1993.

10. Auguste Comte and Italy

Originally published as "L'Italia è meglio disunita," *La Repubblica*, June 21, 1994.

11. Variations on the Theme of a Painting by Poussin

Originally published as "Due miti e un incesto," *La Repubblica*, December 29, 1994.

12. Female Sexuality and the Origin of Society

Originally published as "Quell'intenso profumo di donna," *La Repubblica*, November 3, 1995.

13. A Lesson in Wisdom from Mad Cows

Originally published as "La mucca è pazza e un po' cannibale," *La Repubblica*, November 24, 1996.

14. The Return of the Maternal Uncle

Originally published as "Quei parenti così arcaici," *La Repubblica*, December 24, 1997.

1. "Full Text of Earl Spencer's Funeral Oration," *BBC*, http://www.bbc
.co.uk/news/special/politics97/diana/spencerfull.html.
2. Cai Hua, *A Society Without Husbands or Fathers: The Na of China*, trans.
Asti Hustvedt (New York: Zone, 2000).

15. Proof by New Myth

Originally published as "I miti: uno sguardo dentro la loro origine," *La Repubblica*, April 16, 1999.

16. *Corsi e ricorsi:* In Vico's Wake

Originally published as "Gli uomini visti da un'ameba," *La Repubblica*, March 9, 2000.

1. D. Wilson, "Human Population Structure in the Modern World: A Malthusian Malignancy," *Anthropology Today* 15, no. 6 (December 1999): 24.
2. *The New Science of Giambattista Vico*, trans. from the 3rd ed. (1744) by Thomas Goddard Bergin and Max Harold Fisch (Ithaca, NY: Cornell University Press, 1948), book 1, sec. 4, para. 349, p. 20, https://archive .org/stream/newscienceofgiam030174mbp/newscienceofgiam030174 mbp_djvu.txt.

INDEX

assonance, 96–97, 127
astrophysics, 77
Aztecs, 74

Bacon, Francis, 137
Balzac, Honoré de, 46
Baudelaire, Charles, 100, 101
biological evolution, 30
biological kinship, 46
biological parents, 43–45
biological paternity, 43, 45
bipartite ideology, 56
bipartitions, 52, 53
birds, colors of, origin of, 130, 131
blade industries, 28
Boas, Franz, 67
Bohr, Niels, 81
Bororo, 60, 62
Brazil, 36, 37, 38, 51, 53, 54, 60, 61, 73, 74, 87
bûche de Noël, 7
Buffon, Georges-Louis Leclerc, Comte du, 47

Calvinism, 91
cannibalism, 85, 86–89, 113–14
carnivores, 114, 115, 116, 117
carnivorous diets, 113, 114
casting out nines (*preuve par neuf*), 131
Castor, 52
Catholicism, 91, 93, 97
chained rhymes, 127
Chamberlain, Basil Hall, 21, 22
Chéruel, Pierre Adolphe, 7
children, role of, 15, 16

Christmas: celebrations of in United States, 4; church criticism of, 18; contradictory characteristics of, 16; development of celebration in France, 5, 6; as gathering together and communion, 13; non-Christian aspects of, 13; as opposition between children and adults, 12, 15; as opposition between dead and living, 12; as rhythm of increased solidarity and exacerbated antagonism, 14
Christmas begging, 15
Christmas trees, 6, 7–8
chronophotography, 58
clay, origin of, 129, 131
closed crowns, 58, 59
Comte, Auguste, 90–98, 115, 116
concatenated rhymes, 127
consanguinity, 123
copper, 62–63
corsi e ricorsi, 137, 138
Cosmographie universelle [*Universal Cosmography*] (Thevet), 53
Coyote, 51
Creutzfeldt-Jakob disease, 84, 85, 87, 113, 114
crowns, 58, 59
culture, transition from nature to, 107
cyclical adenosine monophosphate, 136

Dante. *See* Alighieri, Dante
death, relationships with, 17
demiurge, 52, 53
Democriticus, 80

Désaugiers, Marc-Antoine, 51

Descartes, René, 76

Dictionnaire historique des institutions, moeurs et coutumes de la France [*Historical Dictionary of Institutions, Mores, and Customs of France*], 7

diffusion, 5, 6, 36

Discourse on the Origin of Inequality (Rousseau), 74

diseases: Creutzfeldt-Jakob, 84, 85, 87, 113, 114; kuru, 83–86, 87, 113; mad cow, 84, 113, 114, 117, 118, 119

domestication of animals, 33, 34, 35, 36, 133

domestic cell, 125

dualism, 16, 56

duality, 11, 78, 79

Dumézil, Georges, 56

du Tillot, Guillaume, 13

eccentric avant-garde, 98

Echo (figure in myth), 99, 100, 101–2, 104

echo, 99–100, 103, 104

Echo and Narcissus [*The Death of Narcissus*] (Poussin), 99, 104

empiricism, 110

endocannibalism, 87, 113

Enlightenment, 74, 91

Essais (Montaigne), 73, 75

estrus, disappearance of/loss of, 107–8, 109, 111

ethnologists: appeal of jewelry to, 57–63; as being thrust onto public stage, 42; Bohr's invitation for

contemporaries to turn to, 81; changing role/research behaviors of, 38; as consultant, 47–48; hiring of by tribes, 38; lawyers as turning to, 39; on medically assisted reproduction, 44, 47; problems raised by as not disappearing but rather shifting, 47, 48; as seeing great variety of individual behaviors in all societies, 41; wariness of indigenous minorities toward, 38

ethnology, as seen as last incarnation of colonialism, 37

evolution: biological evolution, 30; macroevolution, 30; as not one type of, 30; regressive evolution, 32; of species as coming about slowly and gradually, 30; technological evolution, 30

exocannibalism, 87

explanation, types of, 134

external differences, clashes between, 48

external rigidity, 25

factory farming, 116

Father Christmas, 7, 8, 12

Father Flog, 2, 9

female sexuality, and origin of society, 105–11

feminist movements, 106

fetishism, 95

fieldwork, transformation of, 38

figurative language, 81

fishers, 113

flake-based industries, 28

fog, origin myth of, 49–51
foreign customs, adoption of, 6
formal homology, 137
fosterage, 122
France: celebrations of Christmas
    in, 4, 5, 6; reconciliation between
    public and religion in, 3
France-Soir, 1–2, 3
fraternized rhymes, 127
Frazer, James George, 18
Furetière, Antoine, 100

Gajdusek, Carleton, 83–84
gender studies, 106
generalized sexual commerce, 108
genetic code, 135, 138
genetic inheritance, 135
ghost marriages, 45
gold, 59, 61, 62
goldsmithery, 59
Gómez-Imbert, Elsa, 128
grain production, 117
Greek philosophy, 79
Greeks, 101, 102, 103, 104
Grimes Cave (England), 29

Haida Indians, 67
heraldic symbols, 58
herbivores, 115, 116
Herodotus, 21
Hértier-Augé, Françoise, 44
Histoire de Lynx [*The Story of Lynx*] (Lévi-
    Strauss), 49, 55, 56
Hobbes, Thomas, 73, 137
homelands, 92
Homo erectus, 111, 136

Homo habilis, 110, 111, 136
Homo sapiens, 110, 136
Homo sapiens sapiens, 30
Horace, 12
human beings: eating preferences of,
    113; relationships of with animals,
    115; and their works, 71
human body, substances drawn from,
    86, 88
human brain matter, 85, 88, 114
human females, compared to other
    female mammals, 106–7
Humanity (Comte), 94–95, 96
hunter-gatherers: as believing life
    is better without agriculture, 34;
    productivity rate of, 32; reasons for
    not needing/wishing to cultivate
    land and raise livestock, 33
hunters, 113

identity, principle of, 77
imperial crown, 59
imperial power, divine origin of, 25
Incas, 74
incest, 103, 108, 123, 125
Indians: distinction between Indians
    and whites, 53–54; welcoming
    attitude of toward whites, 54, 56.
    See also specific Indian tribes
indigenous minorities, ethnic identity
    and moral/legal rights of, 37
intertribal fairs, 29
Inuit, 101
invariant relationships, 57
Iroquois, 78
Italian Renaissance, 98

tetracalcium phosphate, 35

Thevet, André, 53

Things Japanese (Chamberlain), 21

Thompson, D'Arcy Wentworth, 57, 58

Tlingit, 69–70, 71

tool handling, 22, 23, 24

traditional morality, and advances of science, 47

transmutation, 115–116

Tsimshian Indians, 67, 70

Tupinamba, origin myth, 53

twinship, 52–53, 78

United States, influence and prestige of on French Christmas celebrations, 4

vegetarian diets, 113, 118

verbal code, 135, 136

Vico, Giambattista, 81, 82, 137, 138

Voltairean deism, 91

weapons, stone imitations of metal weapons, 29

Western thought, 23–24

whites: distinction between whites and Indians, 53–54; motivations of toward Indians, 56

wind, origin myth of, 49–51

writing, appearance of, 29

Yanomami Indians, 87

Yule log, 7

ABOUT THE AUTHOR

Claude Lévi-Strauss was born in Brussels on November 28, 1908. He held the chair of social anthropology at the Collège de France from 1959 to 1982 and was elected a member of the Académie Française in 1973. He died in Paris on October 30, 2009.

Among his works:

La vie familiale et sociale des Indiens Nambikwara. Paris: Société des Américanistes, 1948. [*Family and Social Life of the Nambikwara Indians.* Trans. Eileen Sittler. New Haven, Conn.: Human Relations Area Files, 197?]

Les structures élémentaires de la parenté. Paris: Presses Universitaires de France, 1949; The Hague: Mouton, 1967. [*The Elementary Structures of Kinship.* Trans. James Harle Bell, John Richard von Sturmer, and Rodney Needham. Boston: Beacon, 1969.]

Race et histoire. Paris: UNESCO, 1952. [*Race and History.* Paris: UNESCO, 1952.]

Tristes tropiques. Paris: Plon, 1955. [*Tristes Tropiques.* Trans. John Russell. New York: Atheneum, 1961.]

Anthropologie structurale. Paris: Plon, 1958. [*Structural Anthropology.* Trans. Claire Jacobson and Brooke Grundefest Schoepf. New York: Basic Books, 1963.]

Le totémisme aujourd'hui. Paris: Presses Universitaires de France, 1962. [*Totemism.* Trans. Rodney Needham. Boston: Beacon, 1963.]

La pensée sauvage. Paris: Plon, 1962. [*The Savage Mind.* Chicago: University of Chicago Press, 1966.]

Mythologiques. Paris: Plon, 1964–1971. Vol. 1, *Le cru et le cuit.* Vol. 2, *Du miel aux cendres.* Vol. 3, *L'origine des manières de table.* Vol. 4, *L'homme nu.* [*Introduction to the Study of Mythology.* Trans. John Weightman and Doreen Weightman. New York: Harper & Row, 1969–1981. Vol. 1, *The Raw and the Cooked.* Vol. 2, *From Honey to Ashes.* Vol. 3, *The Origin of Table Manners.* Vol. 4, *The Naked Man.*]

Anthropologie structurale II. Paris: Plon, 1973. [*Structural Anthropology II.* Trans. Monique Layton. Harmondsworth, U.K.: Penguin, 1973.]

La voie des masques. Geneva: Albert Skira, 2 vols. 1975; rev., augmented ed. followed by *Trois excursions.* Paris: Plon, 1979. [*The Way of the Masks.* Trans. Sylvia Modelsky. Seattle: University of Washington Press, 1982.]

Le regard éloigné. Paris: Plon, 1983. [*The View from Afar.* Trans. Joachim Neugroschel and Phoebe Hoss. New York: Basic Books, 1985.]

Paroles données. Paris: Plon, 1984. [*Anthropology and Myth: Lectures, 1951–1982.* Trans. Roy Willis. New York: Blackwell, 1987.]

La potière jalouse. Paris: Plon, 1985. [*The Jealous Potter.* Trans. Bénédicte Chorier. Chicago: University of Chicago Press, 1988.]

Histoire de lynx. Paris: Plon, 1991. [*The Story of Lynx.* Trans. Catherine Tihanyi. Chicago: University of Chicago Press, 1995.]

Regarder écouter lire. Paris: Plon, 1993. [*Look, Listen, Read.* Trans. Brian C. J. Singer. New York: Basic Books, 1997.]

Saudades do Brasil. Paris: Plon, 1994. [*Saudades do Brasil: A Photographic Memoir.* Trans. Sylvia Modelski. Seattle: University of Washington Press, 1995.]

Oeuvres. Paris: Gallimard, 2008.

L'anthropologie face aux problèmes du monde moderne. Paris: Seuil, 2011. [*Anthropology Confronts the Problems of the Modern World.* Trans. Jane Marie Todd. Cambridge, Mass.: Harvard University Press, 2013.]

L'autre face de la lune: Écrits sur le Japon. Paris: Seuil, 2011. [*The Other Face of the Moon.* Trans. Jane Marie Todd. Cambridge, Mass.: Harvard University Press, 2013.]

Gilles Deleuze, *Nietzsche and Philosophy*

David Carroll, *The States of "Theory"*

Gilles Deleuze, *The Logic of Sense*

Julia Kristeva, *Strangers to Ourselves*

Alain Finkielkraut, *Remembering in Vain: The Klaus Barbie Trial and Crimes Against Humanity*

Pierre Vidal-Naquet, *Assassins of Memory: Essays on the Denial of the Holocaust*

Julia Kristeva, *Nations Without Nationalism*

Theodor W. Adorno, *Notes to Literature*, vols. 1 and 2

Richard Wolin, ed., *The Heidegger Controversy*

Hugo Ball, *Critique of the German Intelligentsia*

Pierre Bourdieu, *The Field of Cultural Production*

Karl Heinz Bohrer, *Suddenness: On the Moment of Aesthetic Appearance*

Gilles Deleuze, *Difference and Repetition*

Gilles Deleuze and Félix Guattari, *What Is Philosophy?*

Alain Finkielkraut, *The Defeat of the Mind*

Jacques LeGoff, *History and Memory*

Antonio Gramsci, *Prison Notebooks*, vols. 1, 2, and 3

Ross Mitchell Guberman, *Julia Kristeva Interviews*

Julia Kristeva, *Time and Sense: Proust and the Experience of Literature*

Elisabeth Badinter, *XY: On Masculine Identity*

Gilles Deleuze, *Negotiations, 1972–1990*

Julia Kristeva, *New Maladies of the Soul*

Norbert Elias, *The Germans*

Elisabeth Roudinesco, *Jacques Lacan: His Life and Work*

Paul Ricoeur, *Critique and Conviction: Conversations with François Azouvi and Marc de Launay*

Pierre Vidal-Naquet, *The Jews: History, Memory, and the Present*

Karl Löwith, *Martin Heidegger and European Nihilism*

Pierre Nora, *Realms of Memory: The Construction of the French Past*

 Vol. 1: *Conflicts and Divisions*

 Vol. 2: *Traditions*

 Vol. 3: *Symbols*

Gianni Vattimo, *Nihilism and Emancipation: Ethics, Politics, and Law*

Hélène Cixous, *Dream I Tell You*

Steve Redhead, *The Jean Baudrillard Reader*

Jean Starobinski, *Enchantment: The Seductress in Opera*

Jacques Derrida, *Geneses, Genealogies, Genres, and Genius: The Secrets of the Archive*

Hélène Cixous, *White Ink: Interviews on Sex, Text, and Politics*

Marta Segarra, ed., *The Portable Cixous*

François Dosse, *Gilles Deleuze and Félix Guattari: Intersecting Lives*

Julia Kristeva, *This Incredible Need to Believe*

François Noudelmann, *The Philosopher's Touch: Sartre, Nietzsche, and Barthes at the Piano*

Antoine de Baecque, *Camera Historica: The Century in Cinema*

Julia Kristeva, *Hatred and Forgiveness*

Roland Barthes, *How to Live Together: Novelistic Simulations of Some Everyday Spaces*

Jean-Louis Flandrin and Massimo Montanari, *Food: A Culinary History*

Georges Vigarello, *The Metamorphoses of Fat: A History of Obesity*

Julia Kristeva, *The Severed Heads: Capital Visions*

Eelco Runia, *Moved by the Past: Discontinuity and Historical Mutation*

François Hartog, *Regimes of Historicity: Presentism and Experiences of Time*

Jacques Le Goff, *Must We Divide History into Periods?*